COMPUTER LITERACY FOR HEALTH CARE PROFESSIONALS

COMPUTER LITERACY FOR HEALTH CARE PROFESSIONALS

Sandra K. Anderson

Delmar Publishers Inc.®

NOTICE TO THE READER

Publisher does not warrant or guarantee any of the products described herein or perform any independent analysis in connection with any of the product information contained herein. Publisher does not assume, and expressly disclaims, any obligation to obtain and include information other than that provided to it by the manufacturer.

The reader is expressly warned to consider and adopt all safety precautions that might be indicated by the activities described herein and to avoid all potential hazards. By following the instructions contained herein, the reader willingly assumes all risks in connection with such instructions.

The publisher makes no representations or warranties of any kind, including but not limited to, the warranties of fitness for particular purpose or merchantability, nor are any such representations implied with respect to the material set forth herein, and the publisher takes no responsibility with respect to such material. The publisher shall not be liable for any special, consequential or exemplary damages resulting, in whole or in part, from the readers' use of, or reliance upon, this material.

Cover design by Spiral Design Studio

Delmar Staff
Executive Editor: David Gordon
Administrative Editor: Marion Waldman
Project Editor: Carol Micheli
Production Coordinator: Teresa Luterbach
Art Supervisor: Rita Stevens
Art Coordinator: John Lent
Design Coordinator: Karen Kemp

For information write, Delmar Publishers Inc.
2 Computer Drive West, Box 15-015
Albany, New York 12212

Printed in the United States of America
published simultaneously in Canada
by Nelson Canada,
a division of the The Thomson Corporation

10 9 8 7 6 5 4 3 2

Library of Congress Cataloging-in-Publication Data

Anderson, S. K. (Sandra K.)
Computer literacy for health care professionals / S. K. Anderson.
p. cm
Includes index.
ISBN 0-8273-4171-7 (textbook)
1. Computer literacy. 2. Medical personnel. I. Title.
[DNLM: 1. Computer Literacy. 2. Health Occupations. W 26.5 A549c]
R858.A48 1992
004′ .02461—dc20
DNLM/DLC
for Library of Congress 91-28401
CIP

Contents

DEDICATION

For Julia,
In loving memory,
and for Julia Nicole,
who helps make each new day,
my very best day.

Preface

This textbook is designed to introduce computer technology to students or practicing health care professionals. The text provides fundamental computer terminology while stressing applications that are important to the delivery of health care. The text includes a detailed discussion of both general computer applications (ie., word processing) and specialized applications (ie., computer-assisted tomography) currently in use in the health care industry.

The allied health professional is becoming increasingly dependent on computer applications in practically all phases of their professional lives. Computers are used today in hospital and clinic business applications, patient care applications, and in diagnostics and research. Health care practitioners, therefore, are challenged not only to become skilled within their own particular field but also to be able to use computers to increase their productivity within those fields. The intent of the text is to introduce computer technology in a format that will be of interest to students entering the health care field for the first time and/or to practitioners who are in need of becoming computer literate.

MAJOR FEATURES

The textbook is designed for health care students/professionals and directly addresses the needs of these individuals. The main focus of the text is that its designed for the end-user, the allied health professional, or the student/professional whose main goal is not that of becoming a computer programmer or systems analyst, but who aspires to become an effective member of the health care team. These individuals are interested in increasing productivity in their own highly technical field. Therefore, the text employs examples of current applications of computer technology within their field of interest. The text intends to motivate the student/professional to continue to study a field not directly related to, but unquestionably relevant to, their career endeavors. The intent of the text is to encourage exploration into an area that can result in increased professional rewards.

Computer literacy texts generally have not been designed with a specific professional group of end-users in mind (except perhaps, accountants and financial managers). Although there are countless texts and publications dealing with what computers are and how to use specific applications software, few exist that relate directly to the health profession, with their own unique concerns and considerations. The demands upon a health professional or student entering the health care field are considerable and cannot be ignored when presenting information that is highly technical. The text, therefore, attempts to increase interest and motivation in the reader, targeting the educational goals of the adult learner.

The text contains an extensive glossary of computer terms. Each chapter presents chapter objectives and study/review questions that will aid the student in developing proficiencies. A variety of study questions have been included.

An instructor's manual accompanies the text. The instructor's manual contains the answers to discussion questions in the text and also contains additional questions that may be used in a test environment.

In addition, hands-on training experiences are available through the use of the applications exercises located in one of the appendices in the back of the text. The exercises are structured in a generic fashion so as not to be dependent on any one brand of software.

The exercises are structured to provide learning experiences within the health care delivery area. The applications exercises use examples from the health care industry, maintaining the link between the hands-on activities and the health care field.

The intended audience is the adult learner, either enrolled in a postsecondary or college environment. It will also be appropriate as an in-house training aid for professionals who are not yet computer literate and need additional training to update their professional skills.

TEXT ORGANIZATION

The text has four major sections, focusing on particular aspects of computers and computer systems currently in use in the health care industry. The first section (Chapters 1–3), covers general computer terminology and concepts as applied to the health care field. The chapters in this section lay the foundation for more detailed discussions of health care applications that are covered in later chapters.

The second section (Chapters 4–7), contains chapters on applications such as word processing, spreadsheets, and databases. This section also provides the reader with a chapter on communications and networking, looking at trends in office automation that are of interest.

The third section (Chapters 8–12), examines computer systems in health care facilities, including administrative, clinical and special purpose systems. Discussions of artificial intelligence, expert systems, diagnostics, and direct patient care and treatment applications are covered.

The fourth section (Chapters 13–14), recognizes the importance of the technological impact of computer systems on our society and on how patient care and treatment is accomplished. It discusses computer crime, problems of electronic processing, and the bioethical implications of computer technology in the provision of health care.

The text's organization allows the instructor to choose those chapters most relevant to their curriculum objectives. The discussion of general computer terminology and applications, along with the hands-on exercises, allow for a basic training orientation. The later chapters introduce more advanced concepts that will be of interest to health care professionals. These chapters include introductory discussions of the applications of artificial intelligence and expert systems in the health care industry, as well as discussion and consideration of practical and ethical issues, including computer crime and bioethics.

ACKNOWLEDGMENTS

My thanks to the editors and staff at Delmar publishers for their assistance, particularly Marion Waldman, Health Sciences Editor, who worked with me extensively during the development of the text. Reviewers who assisted with the project in terms of comments and criticisms of the original outline and the first draft include Tom Kober, Doris Thayer, Paula Mitchell, Dr. Rick Boan, Charles Carroll, Kay Turner, Shirley Hoeman, Patricia Suminski, Madeline Olson, Helen Gemeinhardt, and JoAnn Dever. Their suggestions and insights were invaluable.

Several organizations offered their assistance in the form of photographs to illustrate the text. The contributions are certainly appreciated and acknowledged throughout the text.

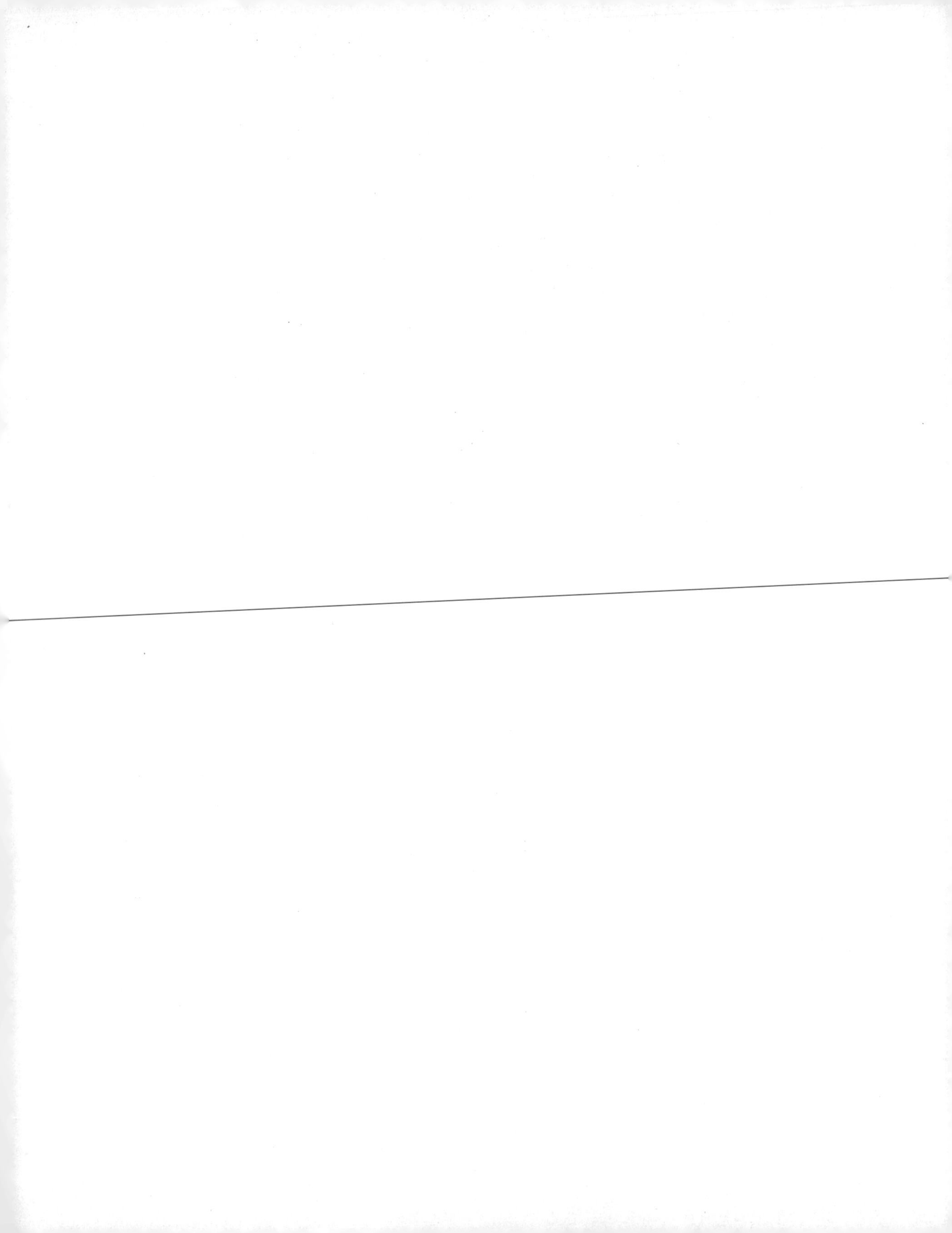

Chapter 1

An Introduction to Computer Literacy

Chapter Outline

OBJECTIVES

1. Define the terms computer and computer system.
2. Identify computer applications within various health care and health-care-related professional settings.
3. Describe the dimensions of computer literacy.
4. Distinguish between the size categories of computers.
5. Distinguish between types of computers based on the type of data they transmit.
6. Define medical informatics.
7. Define computerphobia and technostress.

A GLIMPSE OF TECHNOLOGY OVER GENERATIONS

In the today's fast-paced society, few think back to the days of the doctor traveling many miles to treat a patient—only to have him experience the frustration of knowing that he did not have access to the information or skills needed to help that patient. Today many health care facilities utilize computerized medical information systems to research the latest techniques and solutions available for a specific medical condition—offering to their patients current, life-saving technology.

Applications not even dreamed about in the horse and buggy days, and hardly imagined even twenty years ago, are possible now. Computer-assisted tomography is probably one of the greatest developments in medicine's recent history. This diagnostic technique produces images of organs (such as the heart or the brain) and allows for precise diagnoses, often without exploratory surgery.

Consultations between physicians will occur frequently across channels designed to transmit graphic images as well as textual information. These consultations may occur anywhere in the world in only a matter of minutes and may occur as easily as a telephone conversation occurs today. Medical records and supporting test results will be sent electronically to specialized consultants. These experts will then use computerized systems that analyze the patient information for fast, accurate diagnostic workups, resulting in the administration of appropriate medical procedures. These consultants may even be able to examine the patients periodically during treatment through remote patient observation equipment.

PIONEERING FOR THE FUTURE

Modern technology impacts all our lives. Social scientists predict that the continuing development of computer technology will affect our society profoundly during the next decade. The onset of these changes is evident in the tremendous advances made in the medical field in recent years. Health care providers are increasingly challenged to develop skills by utilizing computer technology as a means of achieving higher levels of productivity during their professional lives.

Allied health professions are expected to grow in the 1990s, creating expanded opportunities for professionals. These opportunities reflect the increased availability of information resulting from computer technologies and related fields. The coming decade in the health care industry will be one of continuing change and challenge. Those individuals interested in pursuing careers within the health professions will be working in a fascinating world of exploration and discovery.

Researchers believe that medical technology has advanced more in the last ten years than in the last hundred. Medical information is accumulating at a faster and faster rate. Professionals are challenged to acquire the necessary skills to process and utilize the information as it becomes available.

Technology is changing our lives. The ethical considerations and choices that we make in the application of new technology will have varied and far reaching implications. In many respects, it will be those who are involved professionally in the use and development of applications today who will determine the benefits of new technology. Professionals entering the health fields need to be aware of the responsibility involved in the many choices awaiting them.

COMPUTER LITERACY FOR HEALTH PROFESSIONALS

To meet the challenge presented to us by increasing information availability, a broad definition of computer literacy will be presented. Basic to this definition is understanding what computers themselves are and what they can accomplish. A **computer** is an electronic device capable of performing calculations and comparisons in a fast and reliable manner. It is designed to allow for the input, manipulation, and storage of data.

Along with being knowledgeable about computers and the terminology related to their use, professionals must be competent in performing data processing tasks by using computer systems. **Computer systems** are a group of components that work together to complete a particular task.

Additionally, computer literate individuals need to be aware of the many social and ethical questions that arise concerning computers and computer systems. Information technology has provided many benefits to our society. However, misuse and abuse of computer technology can and does occur. An awareness of these possibilities aids the professional in protecting organizations and society from their occurrence.

Therefore, mastery within three dimensions determines a **computer literate** individual.

First, understanding what the computer is and the functions it performs. This is a basic requirement for computer literacy. To that end, a basic understanding of terminology and the capabilities of computer systems is required.

Second, performance of basic operations on a computer system in order to complete professional tasks is also a requirement of computer literacy. Being able to use a computer may involve keying in text on a computer keyboard. Or, it may involve more complex operations such as working with programming languages. This text introduces many of the operations and methods currently in use in health care facilities today.

Third, the computer literate individual realizes a social awareness of the impact that computers have on the quality of human life. Significant changes may occur in social structures as a result of computer technology. Realization of the changes that will occur as new technology is introduced can aid individuals professionally by encouraging adaptation to these changes.

COMPUTER APPLICATIONS IN HEALTH CARE TODAY

In any modern health care facility widespread evidence of computer use is readily apparent. In hospital settings, admissions departments process information about new, incoming patients. Using a computer terminal, the hospital representative may enter information about the new patient, including the patient's name, insurance information, and reason for entering the hospital. This information will become permanently stored in the hospital's information system to be retrieved when needed.

Group practice settings or Health Maintenance Organizations submit insurance claims and patient's bills electronically. These claims are "mailed" from a computer terminal. Many other medical offices process bills using a computer system specifically designed for their practice or business. Medical secretaries and administrative assistants set appointments, transcribe medical reports, or use their office computer systems for medical practice accounting.

Many people, when considering the medical field, think only of hospitals or doctor's offices. While exciting opportunities exist in these places, other businesses also provide services directly related to the provision of health care. These businesses contribute to the increasing number of computer applications in health care today. The following sections examine the broad range of professional environments that employ health care professionals with computer knowledge.

Hospitals

Hospital facilities are in the process of becoming automated. That is, they are becoming increasingly dependent on electronic means to perform work. Requirements for those entering the work force of such institutions include an operational understanding of computer systems. For example, medical transcriptionists need to operate a word processor to function effectively within their department. Nursing staffs may need to monitor patients' vital signs using bedside computer terminals. Radiology technicians employ computer technology to gain information about a patient's health status.

Research Facilities

Large research institutions employ many people with a variety of skills. These organizations are often fascinating places to work because they are intimately involved with new developments and discoveries within the health care field. Members of the health care team work together, attempting to find answers to life-threatening questions in such specialties as neurosurgery, endocrinology, and cardiology. Computers aid these research teams in analyzing data and produce information, Figure 1–1.

Physician's Offices

More and more physicians practice medicine with computer assistance. Health care professionals find that using the computer decreases the time they spend at administrative tasks, allowing for more time with patients.

Administrative assistants within a physician's office will need to be computer literate individuals. This person might process insurance claims forms through appropriate entry of patient data into a computer system or might complete correspondence using a word processor.

Insurance Companies

Medical claims companies have a tremendous need for qualified computer operators with specialized medical training. Administrative personnel familiar with large computer systems can analyze information about patient care or aid in processing information for underwriting

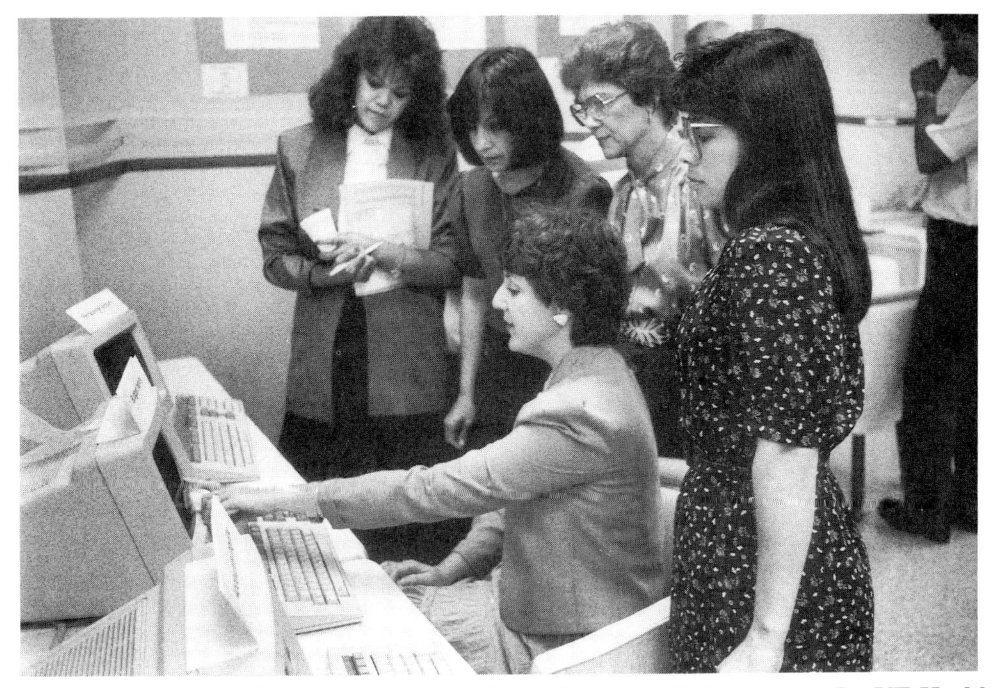

Figure 1–1 Computer classes taught by staff in Information Technology at the UT Health Science Center at San Antonio keep employees and students up to date on the latest hardware and software. ***(Courtesy of University of Texas Health Science Center, San Antonio, Texas,)***

medical insurance. Nurses are frequently employed to review medical records, collecting data that is stored for future use.

Specialized Service Companies

Many types of businesses provide special support services to medical professionals. Examples include companies that manufacture and distribute pharmaceuticals or specialized equipment, such as hospital beds and wheelchairs. These businesses employ administrative and sales staff to help market and distribute their products and use computer technology to increase their productivity.

Specialized Professional Groups

Professional groups that interface with health care personnel also utilize services of individuals with combined medical backgrounds and computer training. Attorneys representing people filing Worker's Compensation claims often have administrative staff who process medical information for them. The computer industry itself offers employment opportunities for personnel with an intimate understanding of the medical environment. These professionals help the computer industry to develop products for more effective utilization by the health care team.

MEDICAL INFORMATICS

The term **medical informatics** refers to the utilization of computer systems technology in relation to medical care and its delivery. Medical informatics, therefore, is an area of study well worth the effort. It involves computers and their abilities and the people within health care environments who use them. Medical informatics analyzes factors that increase the effectiveness of the people who use computers. It also provides a variety of directions for future study that will prove beneficial.

For many years computer systems technology and health care delivery have become increasing interdependent. From the processing of large volumes of insurance claims forms to the diagnosis of disorders, computer systems allow the medical community to provide more services directly to the people who require them.

Today, successful health care professionals are required to be computer literate. The bond between medicine and computer technology has been effectively cemented by the increasingly powerful ability of computers to assist health care professionals in the performance of life sustaining and life saving strategies.

CLASSIFICATIONS OF COMPUTERS AND COMPUTER SYSTEMS

Because computer systems are increasingly commonplace in our hospitals, research facilities, and physicians' offices, they have become an integral part of the health care team. They function to record, process, and store enormous amounts of information.

The types of information that computers record may relate directly to an individual patient: his/her account information, social security number, and even physical attributes such as height, weight and vital signs. Computers might process information regarding the daily progress of a patient undergoing a particular regimen of treatment.

Other types of information may also be processed by computer systems. They can work on complex tasks such as compiling research data for ongoing epidemiological studies or tracking demographic information about particular diseases.

Computer Classifications by Size

Many classification systems exist for computers and computer systems. These include size, type, and function. Manufacturers also create their own classifications through the use of tradenames and available features. Variation in computer size is a frequently used characteristic for differentiating among types of computers.

Computers classified by size can be categorized as supercomputers, mainframe computers, minicomputers, and microcomputers. For the most part, the larger the computer system is the larger its capacity for storage and the faster its data processing ability.

The trend, of course, in new technology is development of greater and greater processing speeds combined with a decrease in physical size. **Smaller** and **faster** are key words in the design of computer systems today.

Supercomputers. Supercomputers are the most complex systems designed and are capable of processing complicated scientific applications. Supercomputers are the fastest, largest, and most expensive of the four classes of computers currently being manufactured.

Relatively few of these systems (approximately one thousand) are operating in the United States right now. However as technology develops we will see an increase in the implementation of these systems. Supercomputers are being operated in research fields, as in the development of artificial intelligence. In addition to the artificial intelligence field, supercomputers contribute to areas like weather forecasting, national defense, and research in health care.

Cray Research and Control Data Corporation are the primary American manufacturers of supercomputers. Hitachi is a main Japanese manufacturer. The development of supercomputer technology in the U.S. is essential to national defense and to the maintenance of a productive economy.

Mainframes. Mainframes are large systems capable of processing massive volumes of data. These computers are basic equipment in hospital environments, insurance claims processing offices, research institutions, banking, government agencies, and large corporations.

Most mainframe computers have faster processing speeds than either the micro or mini computers. There is also greater storage capacity, although current advances are making these distinctions less clear cut. Costs of mainframes vary widely, depending on their processing speeds and storage capacity.

Minicomputers. This category of computer is characterized by larger storage capacity than a microcomputer. It has faster processing speeds for calculations and can support a greater variety of additional equipment. Manufacturers have since developed a "supermini." The supermini computer systems are capable of processing speeds that challenge the performance of a small mainframe.

Manufacturers of mini systems include Hewlett-Packard and Digital Equipment Corporation. The Baxter Technology Group and Cycare Corporation are specialized health care manufacturers. The minicomputers process data in health care facilities in a variety of ways including patient account processing and statistical analysis of research data.

Microcomputers. The last classification considered here is the microcomputer or PC (personal computer). These computers are versatile machines. Since the beginning of the "micro revolution," these relatively small computers have become commonplace in health care settings.

Cost of microcomputer systems can vary greatly. Prices depend on processing speeds and types of additional support equipment such as printers. On the low end scale, the cost of a microcomputer system is less than a thousand dollars. However the cost can go as high as several thousand dollars.

Included in the classification of microcomputers are the laptop and handheld computers, which are small computer systems designed to be portable, Figure 1–2.

College students can use laptops in class to take notes or may carry them to the library for research. Professionals frequently carry laptop computers on business trips or to see clients. Nurses may use handheld computer systems while working on hospital units.

Apple Computer, Inc. is one manufacturer of microcomputers. This corporation has an impressive research and development department that works to bring computer technology to the physically challenged. Other major corporations that manufacture microcomputers include IBM and Datapoint.

Microcomputers are used in health care facilities all over the United States. They can be located in such varied places as large research institutions and world-renowned teaching hospitals as well as in small solo physician practices.

Classifications By Type of Data Transmission

Data can be measured and represented in two ways: discrete and continuous. Discrete data can not be logically divided into smaller units. Continuous data can be divided into infinitely (at least theoretically) smaller units.

Computers are classified according to the type of data they process. Three broad categories exist using this classification system: **analog, digital** and **hybrid.**

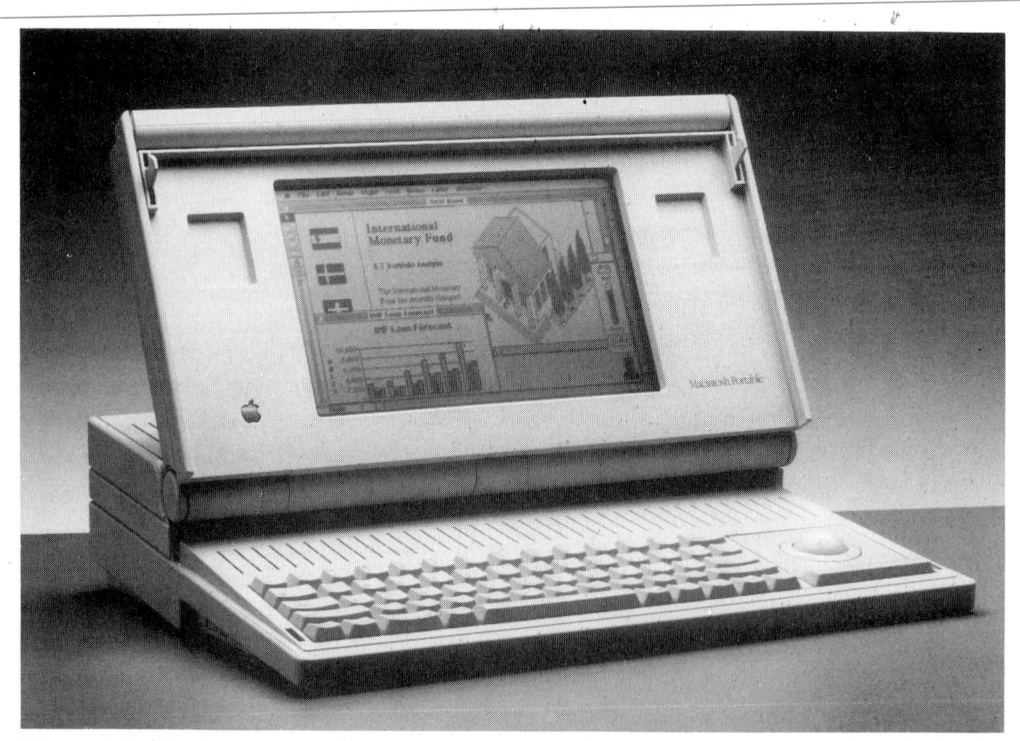

Figure 1–2 Macintosh portable Apple computer *(Courtesy of Apple Computer, Inc.)*

Analog Computers. Analog computers work with continuous data transmission, such as sound waves or volumes. Analog computers process data about measurements. They can process information on various physical or electrical processes involving temperature, voltage, or pressure. For example, an analog computer can analyze blood, measuring for content of substances within a blood sample.

Digital Computers. Digital computers are the most frequently encountered type found in use within the health care industry. Digital computers work with discrete data, using a binary numbering system to represent the data to be processed. Microcomputers are one type of digital computer.

Hybrid Computers. Hybrid computers combine both continuous and discrete types of data transmission. These computers will contain both digital and analog systems, working together to process the required data.

COMPUTERPHOBIA AND TECHNOSTRESS

The term **computerphobia** was coined to describe the symptoms of fear and anxiety people may experience when first faced with the challenge of using a computer. Another term used to describe the anxiety associated with learning and adapting to a new technology is **technostress.**

Professional computer trainers now understand that computerphobia can be managed and overcome. Many, if not most, people experience anxiety when learning new skills. Learning computer skills can provoke anxiety responses or create uncomfortable feelings for people trying to use computers for the first time, Figure 1–3.

TAKE A MOMENT

- ❑ What experience have you had using computers in the past?
- ❑ What are your reasons for studing computers now?
- ❑ Does the idea of working with computers make you feel tension or worry?
- ❑ Do you have any fears concerning your ability to learn how to use a computer?
- ❑ Explore your own attitudes and thoughts about computer literacy. How important is it? Consider both the positive and negative aspects of your thoughts and feelings.
- ❑ There are no right or wrong answers here. Feel free to discuss your ideas with others.

The technology is relatively new; it is not uncommon for individuals to experience discomfort or stress when confronted with change. However, it is important to keep in mind that the rewards of computer skills mastery are exceptional. These machines help people become more creative and more productive professionals.

CHAPTER SUMMARY

The number of health care applications involving the use of computers and computer systems is increasing dramatically. Health care professionals must meet the challenges of the changing health care delivery system by becoming computer literate.

Computers are electronic devices that process information in a fast and reliable manner. Computer systems are functional units that work together to perform data processing tasks.

In order for an individual to be computer literate, they need to define what a computer is, know how to operate a computer in order to perform professional tasks, and be aware of the social and ethical impact that the use of computer technology may have on individuals and society.

Computers can be classified by their size. Supercomputers are the largest computer systems available today. Mainframe computers are large computer systems that can be used to process large volumes of data. Minicomputers are smaller than the mainframe, but still possess relatively large storage capacities and fast processing speeds. Microcomputers are the smallest category and include desktop systems as well as the smaller laptops and handheld computers.

Computers can also be classified by the type of data they process. Analog computers process data that are continuous, such as volumes. Digital computers process discrete data. Hybrid computers are capable of processing both types of data.

People learning to use computers for the first time may experience feelings of fear or anxiety. Terms that express these common reactions include computerphobia, fear of computers, and technostress, the stress experienced when confronted with new technology. Many people experience these feelings but most overcome them and go on to enjoy the experience of using computers.

TERMINOLOGY AND REVIEW EXERCISES

Essential Vocabulary

computer
computer system
computer literacy
medical informatics
supercomputers
mainframe
minicomputer
microcomputer
analog
digital
hybrid
computerphobia
technostress

Review Questions

1. What are the environments in which health care professionals work with computer systems? Are these limited to hospitals, doctor's offices, and clinical laboratories?
2. What is computer literacy? What are the dimensions of computer literacy? Describe the advantages of becoming computer literate.
3. Define a computer and a computer system.
4. Discuss the term medical informatics.
5. Distinguish between the four major size categories of computers.
6. Distinguish between analog, digital, and hybrid computers.
7. Define computerphobia and technostress. Relate your own experiences with these terms.

Chapter 2

Fundamental Components of Computers and Computer Systems

Chapter Outline

OBJECTIVES

1. Identify the elements of a computer system.
2. Define hardware and software.
3. Identify the sections and purpose of the central processing unit.
4. Define peripherals.
5. Identify the major categories of systems software.
6. Identify the five major applications of computer systems.
7. Discuss the considerations involved in purchasing decisions.
8. Define compatibility and describe why it is important.

Computers are categorized by their size and by the type of data that they are capable of processing. Other classifications exist that further define a computer or computer system and clarify the various aspects of the system and the types of processing that it can perform.

In this chapter, elements of a computer system will be presented including a discussion of the major categories of computer hardware and the main types of computer software.

ELEMENTS OF COMPUTER SYSTEMS

Each computer system consists of elements that work together to perform a particular function. Two terms used to identify these elements are hardware and software. Storage may also be considered an element of a computer system, Figure 2–1.

ELEMENTS OF A COMPUTER SYSTEM		
Hardware	**Software**	**Storage**
Central Processing Unit Peripherals	Systems Applications	Diskettes Magnetic Tape Hard Disks

Figure 2–1 Elements of a Computer System

COMPUTER HARDWARE

A computer system's **hardware** refers to the actual physical equipment that is used by the system to process data. Hardware refers to elements of a computer system including the central processing unit and peripheral devices.

The Central Processing Unit

All computer systems, whether mainframe or microcomputers, have a processing unit called the **central processing unit (CPU).** The CPU consists of three main sections: the control section, the arithmetic-logic section, and the primary storage section.

The **control unit** may be viewed as that section of the central processing unit that acts as a department head for the entire computer system. The control unit supervises and manages all the operations that occur within the system. The control section communicates through its circuitry, informing both the arithmetic-logic unit and the primary memory unit of what tasks to perform, and when to begin and end each of these tasks. The control section does not *perform* the actual processing, but oversees its correct completion.

The second section of the CPU, the **arithmetic-logic unit** actually performs processing operations on the entered data. These processing operations can be either arithmetic or logical operations. The arithmetic operations performed are, of course, the mathematical calculations of addition, subtraction, multiplication, and division. The logical operations involve three essential comparisons. These comparisons are based on decisions made by the computer as to whether two values are *greater than, less than,* or *equal to* each other.

The third section we must consider as part of the central processing unit is the **primary storage** or **primary memory** section. This type of memory *stores* data and program instructions; it does not perform any of the logical operations.

Primary **memory** or **storage** may be referred to as simply memory, or it may be called main, or internal, memory. Since different terms have been coined to refer to this particular section of the computer system, it is important to be aware of them and be able to use them interchangeably. Whatever term is used, the functions and characteristics of this section of the computer system remain the same.

Two types of memory are found in primary storage: *random access memory* and *read-only memory.* Random access memory is usually referred to as RAM. One of the most important features of random access memory is that it is volatile or temporary. Once electrical supply is cut off to the primary memory section (such as when you turn off your computer) any data stored within the random access section is lost. If the data that is stored in primary memory will be needed at a later time, it is necessary to save the data by storing it somewhere else, where its continued existence is not dependent on electrical supply.

Read-only memory is termed ROM. Read-only memory, although considered part of primary memory, is not volatile. Read-only memory is installed by the manufacturer of the computer system. It generally gives the computer the basic instructions it needs to start operations. It has characteristics of both hardware and software and is sometimes referred to as firmware for this reason.

Primary storage is measured in bytes, usually in either kilobytes or megabytes. These terms designate the capacity for primary storage to retain data at any time. **Kilobytes** is the smaller of these two measurements with 1K being equivalent to 1024 characters. **Megabytes** is the larger measuring unit and is equivalent to 1,048,576 characters.

Data and program instructions are inputed into primary storage and moved into the arithmetic-logical section for processing. When processing is complete, this data is moved into some type of storage. All operations are supervised and regulated to some degree by the control unit.

Peripherals

Hardware also includes devices required for the input, output, processing, and storage of data. These devices are known as peripherals. Examples of peripherals include mouses, disk drives, keyboards, and printers, Figure 2–2. Joysticks, used for playing computer games, are also a type of hardware peripheral.

Peripherals are a special category of hardware, defined as the physical equipment used together with the computer (the actual processing unit) for performing data processing tasks. Peripherals are devices that are actually plugged into the computer (the CPU) in order to be able to transmit data to it or from it. Frequently used peripherals include monitors and printers.

Peripherals are often classified by the functions that they perform within the computer system itself. They can be hardware specifically designed to perform input functions, output functions, or a combination of both input and output. Consideration of the different types of input and output devices will occur in the next chapter.

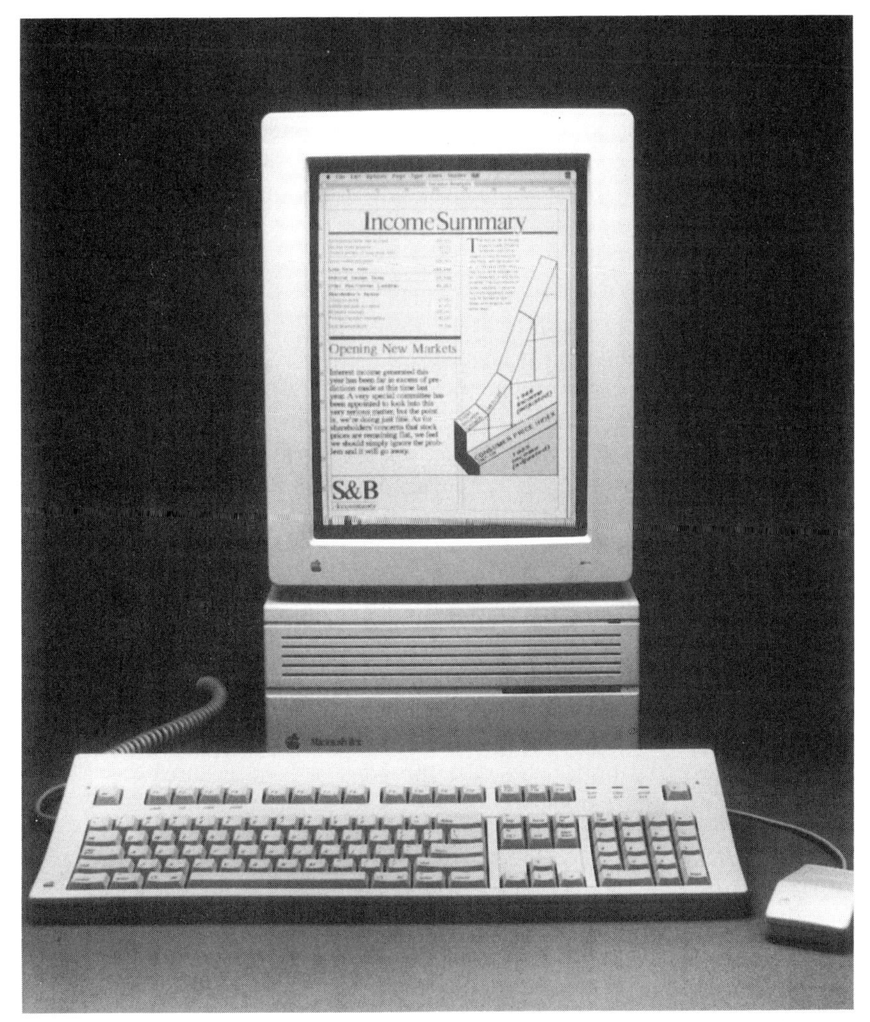

Figure 2–2 Macintosh IICX microcomputer with mouse *(Courtesy of Apple Computer, Inc.)*

Interfacing Peripherals with the CPU

Regardless of the type of input or output devices used, each device must be connected to the central processing unit for data processing operations to occur.

Input and output devices must be connected via ports that link with the computer. There are two types: serial and parallel. Serial and parallel ports are interfacing devices that allow for the passage of data and information to and from input and output units.

A **serial port**, as the name implies, transfers data one piece at a time, sequentially. A **parallel port** will transfer data by groups or chunks. Most microcomputers purchased will come "configured" or built in a certain way—usually with at least one parallel port and one serial port. If more are needed for completion of your data processing tasks, then they must be added to your computer system.

The term **architecture** may be used to describe how the central processing unit and its interrelated elements are structured. An **open ended architecture** refers to a system that allows for expansion at a later date. Expansion slots can be arranged inside the computer housing. This gives the user the advantage of making adjustments to a system as data processing requirements change and increase.

COMPUTER SOFTWARE

Software is simply a set or sets of programmed instructions. Software "tells" the computer hardware what to do in order to complete the required data processing. These instructions are necessary, because without them, the hardware could not complete its processing task. Of course the tasks will vary according to the type of software being used. Software may contain instructions necessary for performing an application, for example, word processing. Other types of instructions, such as those necessary for computing payroll, for example, may also be programmed into software.

However fast processors become or complex hardware systems seem, they are basically electronic machinery that will not operate without the appropriate instructions; the software provides instructions. Software is a computer program or programs: a set or series of instructions written by a computer programmer in order to allow the computer to process data.

There are two basic types of software—systems and applications software. All other software can be categorized under these two broad headings, Figure 2–3.

TYPES OF SOFTWARE	
Systems	**Applications**
• Operating Systems • Translators • Programming Languages	• Word Processing • Spreadsheets • Database Management • Graphics • Communications

Figure 2–3 Types of software

Systems software is concerned mainly with the control and operation of the computer system. It directs, commands, schedules, and oversees the data processing functions to be performed.

Systems software has often been compared to the functions of a traffic control officer directing and supervising the flow of traffic. Similarly, this software has been described as acting as a conductor in a symphony. Under its direction the various parts of the computer system know when to begin and end their performance.

Systems software is grouped into several subdivisions including operating systems, specialized programs such as utilities or translators, and programming languages. Each of these categories provide the computer system with a means of directing and controlling output.

Applications software, on the other hand, refers to prepared programs that perform a specific data processing function for the end user, the person actually operating the computer software. Overall, end users are most likely to use applications programs. On the other hand, computer scientists, programmers, and engineers will be more likely to work extensively with both categories, systems and applications.

Systems Software

Systems software is necessary for the operation and management of a computer system. Three major types of system software are operating systems, translators and utilities, and programming languages. Operating systems are discussed below while information about programming languages is included in an Appendix. Translators and utilities are specialized programs used in advanced applications and will not be covered in this text.

Operating Systems. Operating systems are a set or collection of specialized programs that perform important functions for control of the computer system. Operating system programs interface and communicate between the applications programs, end users, and the computer hardware. Because communication must occur between each of these elements, they must be compatible (capable of transferring data from one another—i.e., from the hardware to the software). Different processors (CPUs) "communicate" with different operating systems. However, all processors do not communicate with all operating systems.

Operating systems for microcomputers. When microcomputers first began to appear on the market, each manufacturer developed their own operating systems for their computer systems. Virtually every manufacturer had a different operating system.

Basically, each computer system must have an operating system in order to function. The different computer manufacturers have not entirely agreed on an industry standard and various operating systems are still being produced and marketed. However, there are several operating systems in use today that are gaining wide acceptance among the various manufacturers.

- **MS-DOS.** The Microsoft Corporation's-Disk Operating System is the most commonly used operating system for microcomputers. It has, in fact, become the accepted "standard" among micro users and is relatively easy to learn and to use. Most microcomputers today operate with the MS-DOS software.
- **Unix.** Unix is another operating system, manufactured by Bell Laboratories. This system may operate on minicomputers, mainframes, or micros. Both Unix and MS-DOS are labeled "generic" operating systems because they work with computer hardware produced by different manufacturers. Unix has been a popular system because of its multiuser (more than one) capability. Unix has also been used frequently in health care settings.

- **OS/2.** IBM and the Microsoft Corporation produce and market a new operating system called OS/2. It promises to be an important system which may eventually replace MS-DOS as the standard for micros. This transition, however, will not occur overnight. End users are just becoming comfortable with the MS-DOS environment and will not be willing to adopt another until it becomes clear that the newer OS/2 will significantly increase their productivity. One of the most important features of the OS/2 operating system is its multitasking capability. Multitasking allows the end user to move from one application to another, working on more than one processing task.

Applications Software

Applications software is the second major type of software; it is software that performs a specific function or functions. It is generally prewritten and prepackaged, although applications software can be developed in-house in order to meet a particular organizations' needs.

One visit to a retail computer software company will give you a good understanding of just how many types of applications software are available for purchase. Accounting packages, computer games, educational packages, and medical management software are all examples of applications software. Applications software is a multibillion dollar industry that is still in its infancy. Because of the seemingly unlimited variety of packages available, it becomes useful to categorize these packages by the functions that they perform.

Overall, there are five basic types of applications software: word processing, spreadsheets, data base systems, communication systems, and graphics. Although the applications overlap somewhat in their functions, this categorization is descriptive of the main function of a software package.

When applications programs contain the capabilities of performing operations in more than one category, the software may be referred to as an **integrated software package**. Integrated software is becoming more commonplace and there are several well known packages that perform more than one application quite well.

Microsoft, Inc., the producers of MS-DOS, have introduced an integrated package called Microsoft Works. Another well known integrated system is produced by Ashton-Tate; it is called Framework. Both Works and Framework have word processing capabilities as well as some database and spreadsheet capabilities.

One of the main advantages of integrated software packages is the ability of the different functions to be linked or merged. For example, a spreadsheet could be placed *inside* a textual report produced by the word processing application. The most common disadvantage cited for the integrated systems is that many of the specialized features available in **stand-alone** packages (packages with only one application) are lost. For this reason, many users still prefer to work with the single application package.

Desktop publishing software is generally an integrated software that performs both word processing and graphics functions. An example of desktop publishing software includes Xerox's Ventura, one of the highest sellers of desktop publishing software. Another popular version of this type of software is produced by Aldus Corporation and is named Pagemaker.

Word Processing. Word processing packages allow the user to format and edit documents on the screen, making corrections as needed before the document is stored or printed. This particular application is one of the most popular and widely used. Numerous word processing packages are on the market and vary in capabilities and features.

WordPerfect, produced by the WordPerfect Corporation, is probably one of the most distinguished in terms of the number of available options. PfS: First Choice is another word processing package that is easy to learn and capable of producing standard textual documents.

Spreadsheets. Spreadsheets are commonly referred to as "number crunchers" because of their mathematical processing capabilities. Computer systems using spreadsheet software can literally perform mathematical operations on hundreds (or thousands) of numbers in relatively short periods of time. Spreadsheet software allows for this type of mathematical processing operation and performs this function quickly and accurately. Lotus 1-2-3, produced by the Lotus Corporation, is still one of the major producers of spreadsheet packages.

Database Management. Database management software allows for the manipulation of data within the data base (a collection of related information). Creation and editing capabilities, sorting capabilities, and comparing and summarizing activities are all considered common data base functions. An example of a database program is dBase, produced by the Ashton-Tate Corporation.

Communications. Communications software allows for the transfer of data from one system to another. This software may allow the user to access information utilities such as CompuServe. Communications software also connects with electronic bulletin boards or mail services, or even provides linkage with larger computer systems.

Graphics. Graphics software allows for the user to create pictorial representations. Business graphics packages allow the user to produce bar graphs, line graphs, pie charts, and other designs that might be used in business presentations. Other graphics packages may allow for more complex, creative designs, including the creation of animated figures.

Choosing Applications Software

The ever expanding selection of prepackaged, prewritten software is, for the most part, quite capable of fulfilling our daily data processing needs. Computer end users want a tool that will make completion of their daily professional tasks easier. Purchasing decisions need to be made that will meet that end.

Whether acting as a buyer for a complex organization or simply adding computer software to a personal computer system, purchasing software can often be a "buyer beware" situation. A few simple guidelines can help the buyer steer clear of some of the hazards along the way.

1. **Find a sales representative worthy of trust.** Because of the boom in the computer industry, many people working in computer sales may not have the experience necessary to make the best decisions. Do not assume that because they sell

computer equipment and software they know everything there is to know. Ask about their computer background and about how long they have worked in computer sales. Even ask for a ballpark figure of how many computer systems they have worked to install.

Once satisfied a sales representative has the expertise necessary, look for other qualities as well. If the sales representative has little patience with your questions before the sale, it's virtually GUARANTEED they won't have any at all once the sale has been made. A willing to help attitude is an essential characteristic in a good sales representative. It is important not be overwhelmed by a sales representative that is trying to impress with his knowledge of computer terminology. Ask the representative what they mean by terms that are not understood. Keep on asking questions whenever necessary.

2. **Identify work objectives.** If choosing a word processing package for preparing general correspondence, first determine your need for any of its specialized features, for example, graphics capabilities. These features may cost more or may not be needed. An accounting office may find math capabilities in a word processing package useful but a student working on class assignments may not use that feature.
3. **Set a price range.** Once objectives have been set the number of packages from which to choose will have narrowed down considerably. It's easy to become overwhelmed with all the "razzle dazzle" and "neat tricks" that some packages can perform. The end result may be overbuying both in terms of price and in terms of effectively meeting your professional needs. A higher price tag in the software industry does not always translate into a better, more reliable product.
4. **Support, support, support.** Before buying a software package find out whether telephone support is available and whether or not there is an additional cost involved for continued access to it. Some companies do not offer any telephone support via 800 numbers; some do, but charge a fee.

   The best situation, especially for new users, is telephone support with no service charge. If choosing to pay for additional support, calculate that expense into the price of the software. If buying for an organization, additional support on a fee basis may prove very expensive. Consider these costs when calculating business operating expenses.
5. **Choose software first.** If buying a complete system, then a good rule of thumb is to choose software first. Once this choice has been made, it will clarify hardware requirements considerably. If computer hardware has already been purchased, then care must be exercised to determine whether the software is compatible. Is there enough memory to run the package? Will your printer or output devices run correctly with the software? Does your software run on your operating system?

   The number of times a particular software package has been modified and upgraded is reflected in the version number on the software. For example, a change from 1.0 to 2.0 reflects major modification to the second version of the program. A change from 2.1 to 2.2 expresses smaller modifications and corrections of software problems in the second version of the software package. A version number of 1.0 indicates that a brand new software package is being introduced for the first time. Version numbers higher than 1.0 reflect the number of times the software package has been modified. A version number of 5.0, for example, is suggestive of a package that has been revised and improved significantly.

Individual pieces of equipment, alone, are not capable of performing data processing tasks. Hardware (both the processing unit and peripherals) together with software, must work as a unit in order to function as a computer system.

Compatibility Issues

Compatibility is a computer *buzzword.* People use it frequently without really understanding what is meant by the term. It is important to understand all the ins and outs involved in working with compatibility issues. The term compatibility refers to the ability to work together. That capacity would seem to be a straightforward requirement but, in reality, it can be confusing when all the variables entering into the compatibility equation are considered.

There are levels of compatibility. One of these levels is **internal compatibility**. This level is the most obvious but problems frequently arise on this level. Internal compatibility refers to the ability of the computer system to work together with ALL of its parts.

Choices for the keyboard (input device), the output device, and the CPU itself must be made. Considerations for secondary storage and for sufficient primary memory must be made. At each step the compatibility issue must be examined, as it directly affects whether or not the computer system will be internally compatible.

For example, does the software support the use of the particular printer chosen? This type of question needs to be answered before the purchase is made, not after the fact.

Another example of a level of internal compatibility might be the need for a graphics card in order to play computer games or produce business graphics and charts. If your software is capable of producing graphics, but your hardware is not, then you have a compatibility problem.

External compatibility refers to the ability of different systems or components of different systems to work together. One frequent problem encountered today is the inability of computer systems to trade data from one system to another without complicated translation equipment and procedures. For large organizations this problem can be an extremely difficult one.

For example, data stored on **floppy disks** of the 5 1/4" variety cannot be used in a computer system that has 3 1/2" disk drives. Disk drives are responsible for the transfer of data from primary memory to secondary storage. The operating systems may be the same but the data cannot be transferred from one system to another easily. These two computer systems are not compatible because of the difference in the type of disk drive they possess.

SECONDARY STORAGE

Because of the temporary nature of primary or random access memory, it is necessary to utilize secondary storage devices. **Secondary storage devices** are physical equipment that allow for permanent storage of data and programs. **Secondary storage** is frequently called **external storage** or **auxiliary storage,** suggesting that the storage device is outside of or external to the main computer elements. While this may be technically correct, it is possible that the secondary storage device is actually located in the same housing as the computer itself. This situation is found frequently in microcomputers that have a hard or fixed disk.

The **hard or fixed disk** is actually a sealed, dust free container which holds a read/write head, an access arm, and a magnetic disk for storage. Because they are contamination free and provide a great deal of storage space, they are a popular feature useful in a data processing environment that requires increased storage capacity. In fact, hard disks are rapidly becoming the standard in microcomputer systems.

Auxiliary storage capacity is increased through means of the fixed disk. Desktop micros often have storage capacities of 10–20 megabytes on up to storage capacities of 120 megabytes of memory. A 10 megabytes hard disk will hold approximately 5000 pages of double-spaced text.

The most common storage medium for microcomputers today is the floppy disk or diskette. The terms disk and diskette are used interchangeably. Floppy disks are magnetic disks with a magnetic oxide coating over a thin slice of plastic. They are considered direct access storage devices.

Floppies, as they may be called, vary in size and storage capacity. The most frequently used are the 5 1/4" diskette and the plastic-encased 3 1/2". Each of these storage devices store data in partitions on the diskette that are referred to as tracks and sectors. Each diskette is divided or partitioned into these sectors and tracks. The storage capacity of the total disk is determined, in part, by the number of sectors or tracks that can be partitioned onto the disk.

Rules for Diskette Care

- Use chemicals such as cleaning solvents and insect repellents with care.
- Do not place heavy objects on top of a diskette.
- Do not bend or fold diskettes.
- Avoid exposure to extreme heat or cold.
- Do not use paper clips on diskettes.
- Use protective jackets to minimize dust and dirt that may damage the diskettes.
- Use felt tip pens to write on diskette labels. The hard points on other pens may damage or destroy the diskettes themselves and the data stored on them.
- Store all diskettes properly in cardboard or plastic storage boxes to protect from dust.
- Do not subject to any magnetic field. (Watch for magnetic paper clipholders, magnetic tape erasers, paper holders, etc.)
- Keep work areas clear of dust, food, beverages, or chemicals that can damage the magnetic surfaces on the diskettes.
- Backup important data.

Other storage mechanisms are used for secondary storage. **Magnetic tape** is one storage device that is used. Magnetic tape is an inexpensive mechanism for secondary storage and offers a high degree of reliability as well as speed and convenience in accessing data and information.

Optical disk storage technologies are currently being developed. These technologies may change the manner in which information is stored. Optical disk storage devices are increasing the amount of data that can be stored on a disk; this feature is its main advantage.

CHAPTER SUMMARY

Elements of computer systems were presented and defined. Computer hardware is one element of a computer system; it refers to the actual physical equipment of the computer system. Computer software is also an element and is a set of instructions that directs the processing the computer performs. Storage is also an element of computer systems.

The central processing unit (CPU) contains an arithmetic-logic unit, a control unit, and primary memory. Primary memory is equivalent to random access memory and its capacity is measured in kilobytes or megabytes.

Computer software is generally divided into two major categories: systems software and applications software. Most end-users are concerned with the use of applications software: word processing, spreadsheets, database management, communications, and graphics software.

Because of the volatile nature of primary memory, secondary storage devices are used as a permanent storage mechanism. These storage devices include hard disks, floppy diskettes, magnetic tape, and a relatively new storage device, referred to as optical storage.

TERMINOLOGY AND REVIEW EXERCISES

Essential Vocabulary

hardware
central processing unit (CPU)
control unit
arithmetic-logic unit
primary storage (primary memory)
memory
storage
byte
peripherals
serial port
parallel port
open ended architecture
architecture
systems software
applications software
integrated software package
stand-alone software
desktop publishing software
internal compatibility
kilobyte
megabyte
software
floppy disk
external compatibility
secondary storage devices
external storage
auxiliary storage
hard or fixed disk
magnetic tape
optical disk storage

True/False

1. Primary and secondary memory are both located within the main memory section of the central processing unit.
2. Twenty megabytes is equal to 20 multiplied by 1024 bytes of data.
3. The control unit of the CPU actually performs data processing operations.
4. External memory is volatile and temporary, dependent on continued electrical supply.

Fill in the Blanks

1. A. ________________ is the equivalent of 1024 bytes. It is designated by the letter ________ .
2. ______________________ are types of hardware that are added to a central processing unit in order to produce either input or output.
3. A set or sets of instructions used by the CPU to perform processing tasks may be termed __________________________ .
4. The section of the CPU that is responsible for arithmetical operations is the ________________________ - ____________________ ________________________ .
5. Auxiliary memory may also be referred to as ____________________ ___________________________ .

Review Questions

1. Describe the sections of the central processing unit and each of their functions within the system.
2. Identify and differentiate between primary and secondary storage.
3. Define hardware and software.
4. Identify the main types of applications software.
5. What is systems software and why is it important?
6. Identify the types of secondary storage available for use on computer systems.

Chapter 3

Data Processing

Chapter Outline

OBJECTIVES

1. Discuss basic concepts related to processing with digital computers.
2. Describe the data processing cycle.
3. Identify various types of data processing as online or offline.
4. Define basic data processing operations.
5. Discuss how data processing operations may be employed in a health care setting.

The elements of a computer system make it possible to perform data processing—turning basic data into different forms of useful information. From the first steps of data collection and input to the final stages of output, a data processing cycle occurs. This chapter will examine methods of data representation, components of the computer system required in the data processing cycle, how data is coded and processed into information, and the basic data processing operations that occur when working with a computer system.

DATA REPRESENTATION

Bits and Bytes

At its most basic level, data, inputed into a computer system, must be represented in a language that the computer can understand and process. Each keystroke that is made by a computer operator must be translated into a machine language before processing can occur. The smallest piece of information that can be processed by a computer is a **binary digit**, generally referred to as a **bit**. A bit can take one of two forms, giving us the term binary. When an electrical charge is present, the bit is ON and takes the value of 1. When no electrical impulse is present, the bit is OFF and this state is represented by 0.

A number of bits are grouped to make a byte, generally in 8-bit units. (Some computers operate on 7-bit units). **Alphabetic**, **numeric**, and **special characters** (such as !, ●,#,$,etc.) require one byte to represent a single character in a machine language. Remember that memory capacity is usually measured in **kilobytes** or **megabytes**. Since a **byte** is equivalent to 1 character, the term 1 kilobyte (K) gives us the capacity necessary to store approximately 1024 characters; 1 megabyte is equivalent to 1000 kilobytes.

Coding

Numerous **machine language** codes have been developed over the years. In order to clarify the relationship of bits to numeric and alphabetic characters, look closely at the three data representations, Figure 3–1.

CHARACTER	MACHINE CODES		
	ASCII	ASCII-8	EBCDIC
1	0110001	01010001	11110001
2	0110010	01010010	11110010
A	1000001	10100001	11000001
B	1000010	10100010	11000010

Figure 3–1 Examples of Machine Codes

ASCII stands for the American Standard Code for Information Interchange and is available in either ASCII-7 or **ASCII-8** bit codes. The ASCII codes are used in microcomputer systems. The 8-bit **EBCDIC** code stands for Extended Binary Coded Decimal Interchange Code. This code is generally used in the larger computers. The code used in any particular instance will vary by the computer hardware requirements.

DATA AND INFORMATION

The raw material, the collection of characters and numbers that are entered into a computer, is commonly referred to as **data**. Data may, of course, vary considerably in terms of content. Basically, however, data represents some type of fact that has been collected.

All data is collected according to some perceived need. On the basis of that need, the data collected will be processed by the computer system and turned into useful information to be analyzed and acted upon. **Information** is the result of data that has been processed in some manner.

After the raw materials or facts are collected, data becomes input for the computer system. In other words, it is entered into the primary memory of the computer system, through means of the input devices.

Processing occurs with the help of the central processing unit. Once processing has been completed, the output or information may be used appropriately. It may be stored in secondary storage for later use or it may be acted upon immediately. Output may also become input for further processing operations. In this way a **data processing cycle** is created.

The same data may be collected and processed into different types of information depending upon the needs of the organization. Basic facts, or data, can be organized in a variety of ways in order to provide useful information.

Suppose, for example, a hospitalized patient requests an item that will result in a charge on their final bill. In a hospital utilizing an automated information system, that purchase is entered into the hospital's computer system together with identifying information about the patient and a catalog number that indicates the item purchased and the price.

Once these basic facts have been added to the computer system, different uses of this basic information may come into play. The accounting department will use the information to update the file on the individual's bill. The central supply section of the hospital may be advised that a depletion in inventory has been made. Further, the purchasing department may use this data to update their files so that reorders of the item may be made. From this example, we can see how the same basic facts can fulfill different informational needs within an organization.

COMPONENTS OF THE DATA PROCESSING CYCLE

Frequently, digital computer systems (those involved in processing discrete data) are defined in terms of the functions they perform within the data processing cycle. Four fundamental components will be presented here. More extensive discussions will occur in later chapters. The four fundamental components of digital computer systems are input, output, processing, and storage, Figure 3–2.

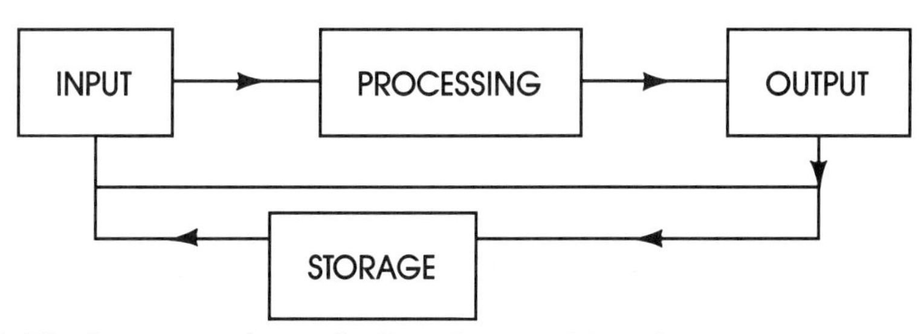

Figure 3–2 The data processing cycle. Data is entered into the computer system, processed in the CPU, and becomes output or information. The output may be stored in secondary storage to be used for other data processing requirements.

Input

All computer systems must be capable of accessing the data to be processed. Therefore, entering data into the computer system or input is required before any processing can occur. Hardware that functions to enter data into the computer system is termed an **input device**. Input devices are generally responsible for translating data into machine readable code. One example of an input device is a microcomputer keyboard used to input characters into the computer system. Another example is optical recognition or scanning devices, such as those used to process price information on the items being purchased at your local grocery store. Optical scanning devices introduced into hospital systems are used as a means of controlling inventory for patient supplies.

Input: Optical Recognition Devices. Optical recognition devices are frequently used to enter data into a computer system. Several different types are available, including optical mark readers, optical bar code recognition devices, and optical character recognition devices. These devices are basically scanners that are capable of discriminating between various input data. One obvious benefit of this type of recognition device is the time saved over keying in the information.

One optical recognition device is known as a **mark reader or scanner**. Mark readers are capable of reading handmade marks on predesigned forms. One of the most familiar applications for this type of device is that of test scoring. Answers to multiple choice or true/false test questions are marked on the special test form by each person taking the exam. Once the tests have been completed they can be passed through the optical mark reader and the final test score can be determined by the computer system.

Quality assessment measurement tools to determine adequacy of patient care on nursing units have been developed, experimentally utilizing the mark reader technology. Answers to various questions about the level of care received are marked on the special test form. Then, productivity scores are developed based upon the answers. These assessment tools are now available commercially and are applicable to a variety of nursing units.

Another optical recognition device is known as a **bar code reader or scanner**. Bar code readers are input devices that recognize bar code product labels. These scanners are typically used in point-of-sale systems at grocery stores. They function to access the cost of products being purchased along with maintaining inventory control information. Some department stores also employ these types of readers using light pens that "read" the merchandise tags.

The last type of optical recognition device is called a **character recognition device**. Character recognition devices are actually capable of "reading" machine printed or handmade characters. These devices are used to process massive volumes of related documents. One example of an application with this type of instrument is the character recognition device used by the United States Postal Service in processing mail by zip code.

Output

Once data has been entered into the computer system and processing has occurred, the resulting information must be accessible to the user. Processed data translated into a final product, or information to be used, is referred to as output. **Output devices** are another form of computer hardware. They are responsible for the transmission of machine coded data into information, which can be interpreted and acted upon by the user. Examples of output devices are monitors and printers.

Printers. One of the most frequently used output devices is the printer. Literally hundreds of printers are available from manufacturers, with a large spectrum of features and price ranges.

Two main categories of printers are **impact** and **nonimpact**. Impact printers actually make contact with the paper surface in order to create an image. Nonimpact printers transfer images without direct physical contact.

Impact Printers. **Dot matrix printers** form letters by impacting small dots onto the paper's surface. These small dots are arranged closely together in order to produce the character on the page. Dot matrix printers are versatile in that they are capable of producing graphic images as well as textual material. Small pin heads forming a matrix actually hit the paper in order to strike the image. The more closely these pin heads are arranged and the more heads that combine to form the matrix, the clearer the printed image will be. Obviously, a print head with nine points of contact will produce an image that is not as clear as one with twenty-four pins or points of contact. Twenty-four pin (or higher) produce print which is referred to as near-letter quality. Dot matrix printers are basically inexpensive. These printers are good choices for when letter quality printing is not a requirement, particularly if the user wants the option of producing graphic images at low cost.

Another type of impact printer is the **daisy wheel printer**. This printer actually "strikes" the desired characters onto the page, in much the same manner as a typewriter. These printers are slower than their dot matrix counterparts. They are not capable of producing graphic images but do produce **letter quality** print. The letter quality daisy wheel type printer is generally a step above the dot matrix in cost and can range from $300–$800 dollars.

Nonimpact printers. If output requirements are such that increased quality printing is desired, then nonimpact printers could be considered. For the most part they are more expensive than either the daisy wheel or dot matrix printers but they extend printing capabilities considerably.

Inkjet and laser printers are considered high end output products for computer systems. They are capable of near typeset quality output and offer varying graphics capabilities. Both laser and inkjet printers would be acceptable choices when establishing a desktop publishing environment. A dot matrix printer might be a good choice for in-house memos and reports or production of continuous feed-forms. The letter quality daisy wheel printer would be used for basic business correspondence that does not require the high print speed, quiet operation, or the near-typeset quality print of the laser.

Inkjet printers shoot out ink in dots onto the paper. One advantage of this printer is its capacity for producing multicolored images. However, laser printers are beginning to introduce color image production capacity.

Laser printers are nonimpact printers that produce output of near typeset quality, operate quietly and can print several pages of material per minute. They are capable of producing graphics and multifonts (typestyles) on a page.

Output: A Look at Voice Synthesizers. If you have ever stood in front of a soda machine, put in your change, and heard the machine respond in an electronic voice "Make your selection, please," then you have experienced what is known as voice synthesization. Voice synthesis is electronic output that imitates human speech.

Researchers have developed the technology of voice synthesizers dramatically within the last few years. Voice synthesizers on the market are capable of reading text appearing on a monitor or even singing a song. Applications for this type of technology range from the manufacture of talking toys to voice synthesis used by businesses for bill collection.

Perhaps one of the most exciting applications for voice synthesis revolves around that of providing hope for speech and/or visually impaired individuals. Speech impaired individuals are now able to use computer technology to communicate with others. First, information is inputed through a keyboard and then transmitted to voice synthesized output across communications channels. Visually impaired individuals may be able to "read" by using electronic devices that take input from printed material and translate the printed material into voice output. Undoubtably, these devices improve the quality of life for handicapped persons.

I/O Devices. Computer hardware that can function or operate as either an input or output device are referred to as Input/Output (I/O) devices. VDTs (video display terminals) and CRTs (cathode ray tube) terminals are considered I/O devices. Terminals consist of a television-like monitor and a keyboard. Terminals can be connected to the main computer system right on a desktop or may be linked in other ways to a larger computer system located elsewhere (possibly in the same building in a separate room or even in a building miles away from the terminal). The monitors reflect output in these units, whereas the input is processed through the keyboard.

Storage

As previously discussed, secondary storage is characterized as a means of permanent or long term data storage. Common storage devices include floppy diskettes, hard disks, or magnetic tapes. These devices hold the output, or processed information. Storage is a part of the data processing cycle. Stored information may become input into the computer system at a later time.

TYPES OF DATA PROCESSING

There are two types of processing: online and offline. **Online processing** occurs through a direct connection between terminals and the computer system. **Offline processing** systems do not provide for this direct communication with the processing unit. Online systems are connected to a processing unit via "on line" terminals for data input, or for receiving output. These online terminals may be a typical video display terminal, CRT, or some other I/O device.

Batch processing is one major type of processing that is generally accomplished through the use of an offline system. Data collected for use in batch processing is stored for use at periodic intervals. For example, a payroll system that used batch processing might collect all the information available on hours worked for all employees before data processing would commence for a particular pay period.

Typically, **source documents** are collected with the basic data recorded on them before this data is entered into the computer system and processing occurs. Batch processing is a useful type of processing for particular applications, such as payroll or billing systems, where information does not need to be readily available.

Advantages of batch processing are that it is relatively inexpensive and also an efficient method for processing large collections of data. The major disadvantage, of course, is that a waiting period may exist before current, updated information is available.

Online processing can be referred to as **real time processing**, **interactive processing**, or **transaction processing**. In this type of processing, there is no waiting period for information since the processing occurs immediately after input. Therefore, output information is more immediately available than in batch processing systems.

Transaction processing inputs and processes transactions in the order the transaction occurs. Immediate feedback to the computer operator is facilitated. This type of processing must be accomplished through online communication with the central processing unit. One disadvantage of transaction or real time processing is that it is expensive. However, when immediate access to current information is required, the expense may not be the major concern.

BASIC DATA PROCESSING OPERATIONS

The arithmetical-logic section of the CPU (central processing unit) is responsible for the actual processing that the computer system accomplishes. Remember that the processing performed by the system occurs through either mathematical calculations or the logical comparisons (being equal to, less than, or greater than). These simple operations allow for the organization of data. The particular manner in which data are manipulated and organized into meaningful information reflects the basic data processing operations that occur. Discussion of basic data processing operations follows.

Calculation

One obvious and simple way data can be manipulated into information is through mathematical calculations. For example, annual sales invoices can be added together to give an accurate assessment of revenues for a specific company. Simple calculations involving addition, subtraction, multiplication, or division can be made quickly and reliably through the use of data processing equipment. Complex scientific formulas can also be involved in this type of operation.

Input

This operation involves entering data into the computer system. We have discussed many of the hardware devices through which data entry input operations are executed. The role input takes in the data processing cycle has also been covered. Regardless of the type of input device used to perform this operation, however, data input must occur before other data processing operations can occur. Often this type of input operation is termed **data entry**.

Output

This operation involves the production of information, organizing the data into a useable form. Examples might include a memo or a monthly sales report. Output may result in a hard copy—printed or permanent material. A soft copy, referring to information reflected on the monitor does not produce a permanent copy, since it is held in volatile primary memory. Output operations are performed by the variety of hardware devices, which have already been presented.

Query or Inquiry

When information needs to be accessed or retrieved from the stored source, another operation occurs. This operation is known as either an **inquiry** or a **query**. Usually, queries are performed simply by keying in a name or ID number associated with the information needing to be accessed. Queries are generally a request for some type of information.

Classification

Generally data needs to be grouped in some way in order to be meaningful and useful. **Classifying** may be defined as organizing data into similar categories. Typically, categories used in classifying may be alphabetical, such as male and female designations of M or F. They may also be numerical, sometimes numerical codes that represent various classifications. An example of a numerical classification system might be CPT codes, which are numerical codes representing medical procedures. They may also be a combination of the two: alphanumerical. An example of an alphanumerical class might be a manufacturers' product number such as EV145, which contains both numbers and letters.

Sorting

A frequently used data processing operation is known as **sorting**. This procedure reflects that data has been arranged in a particular sequence or order. Commonly used sorts may be alphabetical or numerical listings: first to last, or smallest to largest. Sorting is a specialized form of a classification operation.

Update

Data entered into a computer system frequently needs to be modified to reflect current conditions. When this operation occurs it is referred to as **updating** or **revising**. Ordinarily, updating involves adding to or modifying existing information. Examples might include changing an old address to a new one or modifying names to reflect changes in marital status.

Summarize

A data processing operation that reduces data into a more compact and functional form is known as **summarizing**. This operation can digest or condense massive volumes of data, resulting in information output that can be used in some significant manner. Graphic representations of data are a useful mechanism for summarizing data.

Storage

Other data processing operations can occur. Data that is entered into a computer must be stored within the CPU. Both procedural instructions and data must be available for manipulation. Therefore, **storage** within the CPU may be perceived as a basic data processing operation. This type of storage refers to primary memory rather than auxiliary, external, or permanent storage.

Retrieval

When program instructions and data are stored in primary memory, a means of accessing them must be available. Thus retrieval is necessary. **Retrieval** or recovery of the data or program instructions from the CPU should be considered a fundamental data processing task.

DATA PROCESSING OPERATIONS AT WORK

Now let's take a look at how some of these data processing operations might be employed when the doors of a Health Maintenance Organization open to provide another day of patient care.

Our example concerns Health Plus, Inc., a Health Maintenance Organization. Health Plus offers employers in their city a means of providing comprehensive health care to its employees. Health Plus, Inc. prides itself on offering state-of-the-art quality care to their patients. Of course, they have been operating with a computerized patient information system.

Jan Whitmore is the first scheduled patient for the day at Health Plus, Inc. and is seeing a physician in the OB/GYN clinic.

Ms. Whitmore arrives at the reception desk and states her name. The computer operator keys her name into the IS (Information System) and inquires about her appointment. The operator accesses the information needed, smiles, and tells Ms. Whitmore her appointment is with Dr. Evans and is scheduled in the OB/GYN clinic. Ms. Whitmore is given directions to the appropriate waiting area. The operator has completed an inquiry procedure utilizing her patient information computer system.

Following her appointment, Ms. Whitmore is asked to return for a followup visit in four weeks. She requests that her return appointment be with Dr. Evans again. The scheduling secretary retrieves Dr. Evan's appointment schedule for that week from the information system. The secretary modifies the existing file by adding Ms. Whitmore's name to his appointment calendar on Wednesday of that week at 10 A.M. The scheduling secretary has just performed an update operation. Ms. Whitmore thanks her and leaves the building.

While Ms. Whitmore is meeting with Dr. Evans, elsewhere at Health Plus, Inc. administrative staff are working to analyze patient data to ensure the provision of quality care.

During the past six months, sales staff have enrolled several new, rather large businesses as clients. Because of these new additions, the information system is being utilized in a number of ways.

Additions are being entered into the information system concerning enrollees. Each employee's name and identifying information must be added to the computer system. This operation updates its membership files.

Also, a membership report has been generated for analysis. The report provides the administrative staff important facts about its patients. These facts include the patient's sex, age, occupation, and health status. This information has been totaled and summarized for the management team.

Some concern has been expressed over a new trend in the membership population: the large increase in female enrollees. Several of the newly enrolled companies have large numbers of female employees. Management, discussing this change in membership, has decided to consider hiring a new OB/GYN physician for the purpose of handling the influx of female patients. Thus, the data processing operations of classifying and calculating have provided Health Plus, Inc. with the information necessary for effective planning for the provision of care for their patients, Figure 3–3.

TAKE A MOMENT

- ❑ What other data processing operations might be employed by Health Plus, Inc.?
- ❑ Give examples of how this would provide useful information to the organization.

Figure 3–3

CHAPTER SUMMARY

Data represents the raw facts that are entered into the computer system. When processing has been performed and output is available the resulting product is information. Data must be represented in a form that the computer can understand. Digital computers process bits and bytes. Coding occurs at the input stage and translates characters into the machine language that the computer can process.

The data processing cycle refers to each stage of the transformation of data into information. The input stage, often referred to as data entry, occurs when data is first introduced into the computer system. The processing stage refers to the manipulations that the data undergoes in the central processing unit. Output is the final product, information. Storage refers to the process of retaining the information in some kind of permanent form.

Processing takes place in different time frames. With offline processing, the actual processing takes place at intervals so that information is not always current and readily available. Online systems are real time systems in that processing takes place immediately after input so that information is always current and up to date.

Data can be manipulated in many different ways in order to produce the required output. Operations that frequently occur in order to produce information have been categorized and termed data processing operations. These data processing operations include calculations, input, output, query, classifications, sorting, updating, summarizing, storage, and retrieval.

TERMINOLOGY AND REVIEW EXERCISES

Essential Vocabulary

binary digit
bit
alphabetic character
numeric character
special character
byte
kilobyte
megabyte
machine language
ASCII
ASCII-8
EBCDIC
data
information
data processing cycle
input device
mark reader or scanner
bar code reader
bar code scanner
character recognition device
output device
impact printer
nonimpact printer
dot matrix printer
daisy wheel printer
letter quality printer
inkjet and laser printer
online processing
offline processing
batch processing
source document
real-time processing
interactive processing
transaction processing
calculations
data entry
inquiry
query
classifying
sorting
updating
summarizing
storage
retrieval

True/False

1. Special characters refer to numeric codes.
2. One megabyte is equivalent to 10,000 bytes.
3. Generally, 8 bits are grouped to form a byte.
4. Online processing provides a direct connection between terminals and the computer system.
5. A sort organizes data into various categories.

6. Modification of existing data is referred to as updating or revising.
7. Data storage within the CPU is referred to as auxiliary storage.

Fill in the Blanks

1. A ______________ ______________ is the smallest piece of information a computer can process. When an electrical charge is present, then the ________________ ____________ takes the value of 1.
2. Raw facts entered into a computer system are referred to as ______________.
3. Online processing may be referred to as ______________________ or ____________________ ____________________.
4. When an operator keys information into the computer keyboard, this is an input operation also known as _______________ _______________.
5. Reducing data into more functional forms is a data processing operation known as ____________________________.
6. A _______________ _______________ is a document from which data originates.
7. A __________ ________________________ printer does not have direct physical contact with the printing surface.

Review Questions

1. Describe the difference between data and information.
2. Identify the components of the data processing cycle.
3. Define batch and transaction processing. Describe how they differ.
4. List and describe the basic data processing operations.

Chapter 4

Word Processing

Chapter Outline

OBJECTIVES

1. Identify parts and functions of the keyboard.
2. Define the basic functions of a word processor.
3. Discuss specialized features of a word processing package.
4. Define terminology frequently used in word processing.
5. Discuss important objectives in choosing appropriate word processing packages.
6. Discuss the purpose of documentation.

As individuals develop professionally they will be challenged by the large variety of hardware and software, different trade names, manufacturers, and specialized features that are offered. It is important to remember as one is confronted by this bombardment of "technological wizardry" that software and hardware are designed mainly to accomplish a particular task. Of vital importance is the realization that it is the task and the province of the hardware and software to fulfill the job's requirements. The relevant question remains: HOW WELL WILL THE HARDWARE AND SOFTWARE PERFORM THE JOB AT HAND?

This chapter examines the issues involved in utilizing word processing software applications. The configuration of the keyboard, basic word processing functions, advanced features available on some prepackaged word processing systems, and other pertinent issues involved in the purchase and use of word processing systems will be covered.

KEYBOARD BASICS

An essential part of any computer hardware consists of a basic input device such as a keyboard. The keyboard allows the user to input information in the form of characters or commands. This information is stored in the temporary memory section of the computer generally referred to as RAM or random access memory. (Remember RAM memory is volatile. It is not a permanent storage area.)

Although some variation exists in keyboards produced by different manufacturers, basic features are found on most.

The **ESCAPE** key is marked ESC on your keyboard. This key may function in various capacities depending on the software being used. While working with MS-DOS (disk-operating system), this key will enable you to erase a line of text. While working with WordPerfect, it will enable you to repeat a character for a specified number of times.

Cursor control keys are used to control movement within a document. The cursor is a small blinking dash that allows the user to determine the exact location for inputing characters and commands. Cursor movement is controlled by the directional arrow keys located on the right side of the keyboard. They are in combination with a numeric keypad—a configuration of numbers much like that on a calculator.

The *delete key* is located on the bottom row of the numeric keypad and is usually marked DEL. This key will erase or delete characters from a document at the exact placement of the cursor. For example, if your cursor is blinking directly underneath the letter "i" when you press the DEL key, the letter "i" will be removed from the screen. The BACKSPACE key is a directional arrow key located at the end of the row of numeric keys along the top of the keyboard. This key will allow for removal of characters on the screen one space to the left of the cursor. For example, in a screen display with the word "space" typed in and the cursor located at the next space on the line, pressing the BACKSPACE key will allow the last "e" to be removed, leaving on the screen the four letters "spac."

The **ENTER** or **RETURN** key is located at the position of the carriage return on a typewriter. It is usually marked with a return character and sometimes marked with the word ENTER. When using a word processing software package, it is not necessary to press the enter/return after the completion of every line.

Word wrap refers to the process by which your software controls the formatting of your document and "decides" where each line should end. Right margins are determined by the default setting of the software or by another margin setting chosen by the computer operator.

Because of word wrap, it is only necessary to use the enter/return key when you end a paragraph or want to start text on a new line. Word wrap is a feature utilized in word processing software programs.

Function keys are used either in combination or alone to perform various procedures for the end user, such as saving or retrieving a document or setting up formats for a page. Functions keys on the IBM or compatibles are numbered F1 through F10 or F12. They may be located on the left side of the keyboard or may be along the top.

CAPS LOCK is a key that performs the equivalent function of the Shift Lock on a typewriter with some major differences. While the Shift Lock function on a typewriter leaves all keys in their upper case form, the CAPS LOCK does not. The CAPS LOCK shifts all alphabetic characters into an uppercase, but leaves the numeric keys operative. If accustomed to typing on a standard typewriter, using the CAPS LOCK will take some getting used to. The CAPS LOCK key is considered a **toggle key**, meaning that the function a particular key serves is either on or off. When the CAPS LOCK key is pressed down, all alphabetic characters are UPPERCASE, reflecting the fact that the toggle key is on and operating.

The **CTRL** and **ALT keys** are also function keys. They usually work in combination with other keys to perform a word processing function. When using these keys, the CTRL or ALT key is held down. While continuing to press the CTRL or ALT, the additional key is pressed for whichever function is required. The Shift key and other keys also will be used in combination with other keys to perform particular functions.

The **Num Lock** key is used to control the function of the cursor movement and numeric keypad. Pressing the Num Lock key will allow the use of the numeric keypad for inputing numeric values. The Num Lock key also functions to freeze a display when used in combination with the CTRL key.

Scroll Lock may also be labeled Break key on the keyboard. It can be used in combination with the CTRL key to cancel commands.

The **directional tab key** is in the position where the Tab Key is located on a typewriter, the upper left side of the keyboard; it is a key that is usually marked with two directional arrows. This key functions to provide a tab to the right of the left margin. It also will move characters a tab setting outside the left margin if used in combination with the Shift Key. First press and hold the Shift Key down. While that key is being held down, press the Tab Key. The cursor will move into the left margin.

PrtSc stands for Print Screen. There will be times you will want a hard copy of work on the screen. In this situation, use the Ctrl key in combination with the PrtSc to print the lines on the display line by line. When you want to stop printing, then press Ctrl and PrtSc again.

ESSENTIAL WORD PROCESSING FUNCTIONS

It is advisable, when learning word processing, to think in terms of functions and specialized features. **Functions** may be thought of as those basic operations that assist in the completion of the word processing task. Essential operations include saving and retrieving, editing, printing, and formatting. **Features** may be thought of as methods which allow for enhancement of the essential functions. Features relate to style, form, and speed of production. Examples of features might include the ability of the word processing software to produce different size pitch, fonts, or graphics.

Regardless of the specific word processing package used, all word processors allow the user to complete essential functions or operations. These functions include the following items.

Formatting

This function includes methods for setting margins, tabs, line spacing, and other page layout features.

Editing

This function allows for changes to be made within a document. Changes may include inserting or deleting text and copying or moving text.

Printing

This function allows for the page or document to be printed onto paper or other surfaces (such as transparencies). Printing a document produces a hard copy. The soft copy remains on the screen and/or in random access memory until the computer is turned off or the document or page is erased or stored.

Saving

Each document that is produced may be saved in a document file. Sometimes the terms document and file are used interchangeably. However, the term file actually refers to the named location of material saved on a secondary storage device such as a floppy disk. A document file is not the exact equivalent although it is similar. A document file is a collection of related text, figures, and/or graphic displays.

Retrieving

Once a document has been saved to a secondary storage device then it must be retrieved from storage in order to use or process the data. Locating and accessing the file from the storage device is retrieval.

WORD PROCESSING TERMINOLOGY

While all word processing packages provide the basic functions presented in the previous section, a great diversity of other features exist that can range from simple to complex. When choosing a software package for purchase, it is therefore important to consider the needs or objectives of the user. Let's take a look at the variety of features available on the market today.

Modes of Operation

Once text has been entered, it is possible to use a **typeover mode** in order to change text. This is accomplished through moving the cursor to the position at which you wish to make changes, setting the program to the correct mode, and then typing directly over the previously entered text. Another way to change or edit text involves use of the **insert mode**. The insert mode allows for text to be "added" to a document by positioning the cursor in the correct location and then keying in the additional material. Most word processing packages are set with the **insert mode** as the default setting. The **default setting** is that setting that has been chosen by the manufacturer as the standard mode of operation. Default settings also exist for other features such as margins, tabs, pagination, and left and right justification. It is possible to change these default settings by using the appropriate commands.

Block Operations

Block operations may include delete, copy, and moving text. A block operation usually involves more than one character, it may involve a line, a sentence, a page or even twenty pages. The text is marked or highlighted. Once it has been marked or blocked, the text may be modified in the appropriate manner.

Block operations can move or copy text. The **move command** entails marking out a block of text and actually relocating it in another position. Sometimes moving text is referred to as a "cut and paste" operation. After a move operation has been completed, the original block of text is positioned in its new location. The **copy command** involves marking out a block of text and making a copy of the original text to move to a new location. Copying text results in two exact duplicates of text, the original that remains in its original location and the copied text that has been repositioned.

Search Operations

Search procedures can also be considered a block operation. In different instances it might be useful to "look through" a block of text and identify a particular word, phrase, or name. Search operations can identify a block of characters in a single page or in a multipaged document.

Search operations can be used in documents that require minor editing. For example, the search and replace procedure can identify common names that may have been misspelled in a document, allowing for correction by inserting the correct spelling of the name automatically.

OTHER WORD PROCESSING FEATURES

The **on-screen formatting** feature allows for the changes made within a document to be shown on the screen. Manufacturers vary in what they mean when they advertise "on-screen" formatting. Some word processing packages that advertise this feature are not actually capable of performing it.

Pagination refers to the ability of a word processing package to allow for control of page formatting. Many different formats are available. Page numbering may be turned off, may occur on every other page, or may be positioned on the page according to the writer's preference.

Hard and soft page breaks control page positioning. Most word processing systems allow for a certain number of lines per page. If the amount of lines exceeds that limit, then a soft page break will occur at that point. Hard page breaks may be inserted by the individual using the software when the document format requires that text be placed on specific lines within a page.

Headers and footers are page formatting features that allow for pages to be marked in various ways for the purpose of identification. Headers, being placed at the top of the page, may include information like the title, author, and page number of a document. Footers may contain similar information but are located on the bottom of a document page.

Justification is a page formatting feature that allows for alignment of margins. Right justification refers to aligning the right margins so that each line of text will end at the same line space.

Widows and orphans refer to lines of a paragraph that may be improperly positioned due to the default line settings of the software. If a paragraph ends with a single line beginning on a new page, then adjustments may need to be made to accommodate the line on the preceding page. The orphan term refers to the situation where a new paragraph begins on the last line of a page. Again, this situation requires correction. Word processing packages vary in their capabilities for managing these page formatting problems.

A **Status line** will generally inform the end user where exactly they are working in the document, giving information on page location, line number, and space position of the cursor.

Hard and soft returns are page formatting features. When a word processing package marks the end of a line, a soft return is entered into the document. These soft returns will change if text is later inserted or deleted, automatically altering the positioning of the end of a line. Hard returns are used by pressing the ENTER key. This denotes that the line should end at that point. Hard returns are used, for example, to mark the end of a paragraph.

Scrolling allows the computer operator to control the location of the cursor within a document. When working with a lengthy document consisting of several pages, the scrolling feature allows the operator to move quite quickly from one location in the document to another.

Hyphenation of words often requires the use of special combinations of keys in order to insert what is referred to as a **hard hyphen**. A hard hyphen is one that will remain in the word regardless of the position of the word within a line. A **soft hyphen**, on the other hand, may lose its hyphen if its positioning on the line changes. Usually your word processing package will allow for the hyphenation feature to be turned off or on depending on the preference of the user.

ADVANCED WORD PROCESSING APPLICATIONS

Math Features. Some word processing packages offer limited mathematical calculations to be used while working with a document. This specialized feature is useful to those who are working with business estimates, service contracts, billings, or other accounting functions.

Multicolumn Output. Word processing packages often allow for more than one column to be shown on the screen and for each column on the screen to follow its own format in terms of line space. Newspaper print is in a column format as are many company newsletters so this feature can be useful in a variety of settings.

Merge Operations. Mail merge operations are particularly useful word processing applications. Form letters are prepared and reproduced without the necessity of retyping. Group practice settings may use merge operations in mailing out collection letters from delinquent accounts. Information is keyed into the computer system then reproduced with the correct information placed in the proper location on the form.

Macros. Macros are a series of keystrokes that have been saved under a filename which can be used and inserted into a document or documents repeatedly. Macros can be created that will allow the end user to save a closing that is frequently used to end business letters. They can also save functions by calling up the appropriate commands and entering them into a new document. Macros are time-saving devices. When used appropriately they can function to increase production considerably.

Windows. Using windows in a word processing package allows the user to move from one document to another while keeping the documents available on the screen. This application is becoming quite popular.

Spell Checks and Thesaurus. Many word processors offer features which assist an individual in producing quality work. Some of these features are standard and others can be added for use with particular software packages. Standard features include the spelling and thesaurus functions. With the spelling function, it becomes possible to check every word for accuracy within a document. The spell check will mark any word not spelled accurately or any word not found within its dictionary. The spell check is an aid to proofreading and checking for accuracy. However, it is important to remember that the spell check alone will not correct for improper usage of a correctly spelled word. Consider the following examples:

INCORRECT	CORRECT
Its a good hospital.	It's a good hospital.
There doctor is out of town.	Their doctor is out of town.

A spell check will not locate these types of errors so it is important to remember that careful proofreading may still be required.

The thesaurus function can aid a writer when seeking words with similar meanings. If a particular word has been repeated within a document quite often, a computer operator may want to find a word that will aid in improving the writing style. The thesaurus can be quite helpful in this respect.

Supplemental software. Specialized dictionaries and grammar and style checkers are still relatively new on the market and generally are not included in a word processing package. These types of software can be purchased and used to supplement the standard package, Figure 4–1.

Grammar checkers will try to correct for improper usage within a document while style checker functions to review a document for vocabulary appropriateness. For example, a

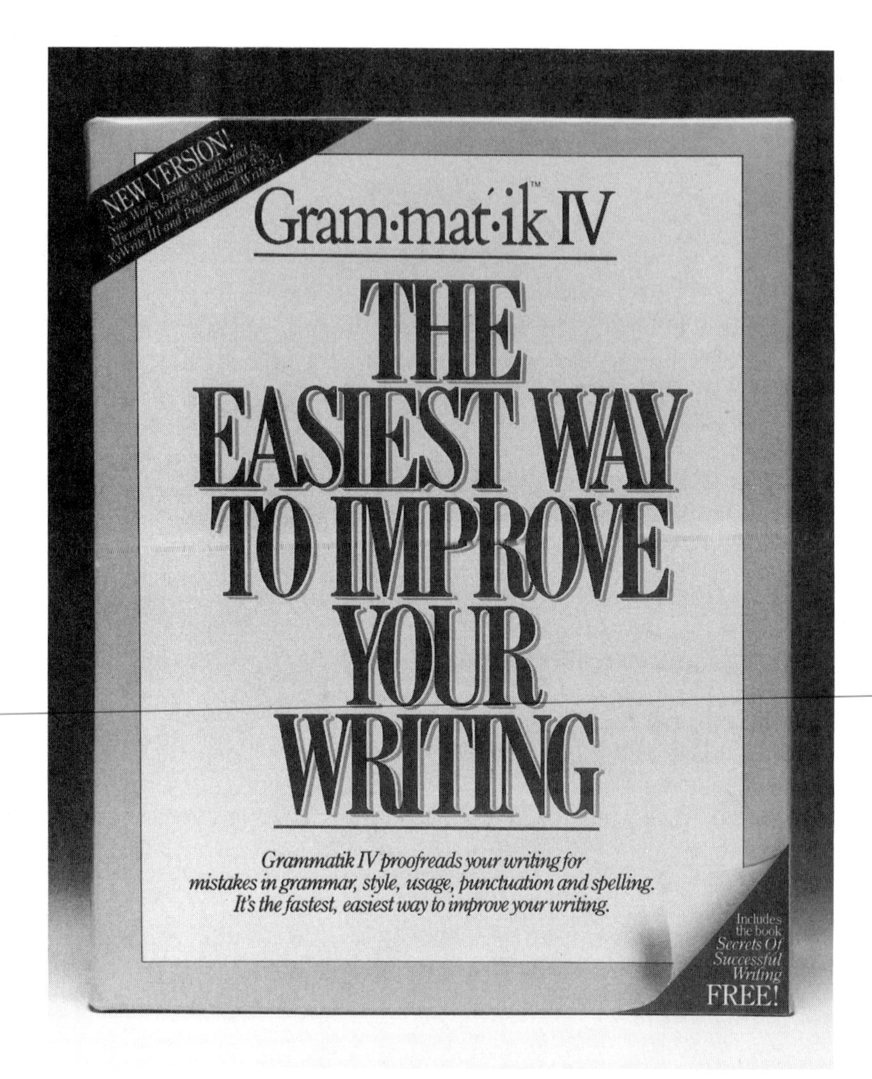

Figure 4–1 Grammatik IV: a grammar checker that proofreads for errors in grammar, style, punctuation, and spelling ***(Courtesy of Reference Software)***

person writing a juvenile fiction novel would want to check the vocabulary of the text to see that it was appropriate for that reading level, Figure 4–2.

Specialized dictionary packages are available for purchase that allow the user to spell check for medical or pharmaceutical terminology. One popular package is Stedman's Medical Dictionary, that offers over 65,000 medical terms in its dictionary, Figure 4–3.

LEARNING WORD PROCESSING

Many of the terms presented in this chapter may seem confusing; however, they become clear in a very short time. Hands-on experience is required to learn how functions and

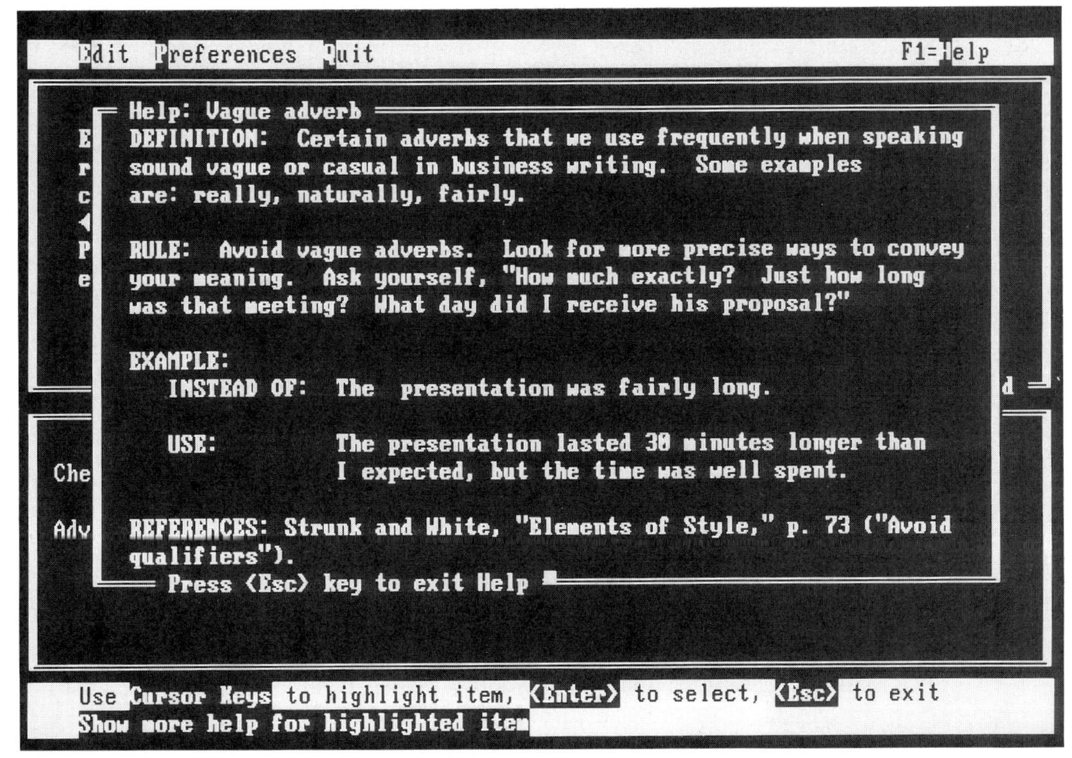

Figure 4–2 Grammatik IV: sample correction screen *(Courtesy of Reference Software)*

features really operate. Reading about terminology can not replace time spent working on a computer using a word processing program. However, with some small investment in time and practice, these terms will seem as familiar as a next door neighbor.

It is important when using a word processing program, or any other applications program for that matter, to remember to make a **backup file**. This backup file is a copy of the work that has been produced. One of the most frustrating experiences of computer operators is that of losing work. This loss of data can occur for a variety of reasons including power failure, power surges, and operator error. While gaining proficiency in using a word processor, continually save work in order to prevent loss of data. The main purpose of creating a backup file is to avoid loss of data. Depending on the importance of the work, it might be necessary to create more than one backup file and to store them in different locations. Accountants that keep records on small businesses for a number of years may, for example, locate one set of backup files in their office and another in their homes to guard against possible loss of valuable data through theft or fire.

USING DOCUMENTATION

Perhaps one of the most difficult tasks in learning to use a computer software package is becoming comfortable with **documentation**. Documentation refers to the written material that accompanies your software when it is purchased. It contains all the information necessary or required to use software appropriately. At times when faced with a task of

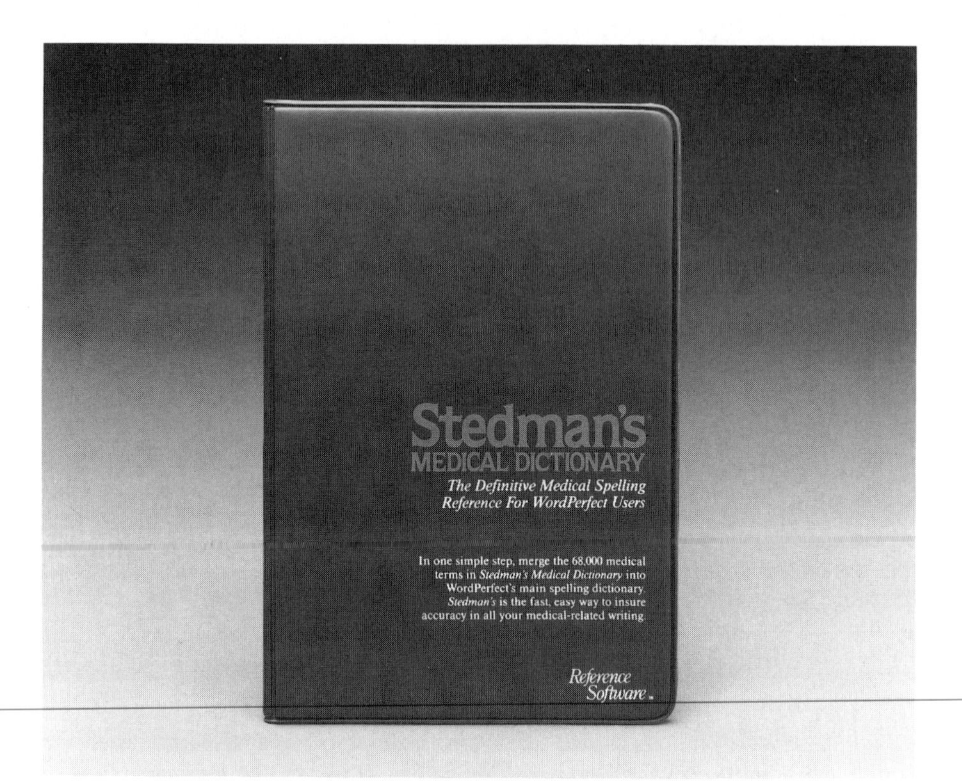

Figure 4–3 Stedman's Medical Dictionary checks medical documents for correct spelling of medical terms ***(Courtesy of Reference Software)***

producing a particular document, it is possible to come across a requirement that is not familiar. If no one is immediately available to answer questions, then it may be necessary to look up the answer in the manufacturer's documentation. Reading and understanding technical material is difficult. However, it will be worth the effort to become comfortable enough to find the answers when needed.

DESKTOP PUBLISHING

Large organizations, such as research institutions or medical training facilities, may have their own printing departments for the production of special documents. Many of these organizations are now using what is referred to as **Desktop Publishing**. Desktop publishing software allows for the production of high quality graphics along with textual information. Most often these documents are produced using a laser printer which prints a near-typeset quality document. The results are impressive.

COMMAND DRIVEN, MENU DRIVEN, AND USER FRIENDLY

Most manufacturers want their software to be easy to use—the easier it is to train someone to use a particular software system, the greater the sales for that system will be. At least, this premise is the philosophy behind producing **user-friendly** software packages. **Menu driven** software is another term often used to imply that a package is relatively simple and straightforward to use. **Command driven** requires the user to use a particular sequence of keys in order to perform a particular operation.

When making decisions on the purchase of software, however, it is important to know the limitations of the software in relation to production objectives. For example if software is going to be used in a scientist's research lab that makes frequent use of equations, using superscripts or subscripts, it is important to chose a word processing package (and appropriate hardware) that is capable of producing the required output in an efficient manner.

WORD PROCESSING AT WORK

Most hospitals and many group practice settings, including Health Maintenance Organizations, have transcription departments, employing individuals with secretarial and specialized medical terminology training.

The transcriptionist is responsible for recording a physician's standard reports such as discharge summaries after hospitalization and surgical summaries describing procedures that were performed. Since these reports or summaries are legal documents, the production of an accurate and complete report is essential. Often there are time restraints imposed on the production of the reports, particularly on those reports dealing with hospitalized patients. The Joint Commission of Hospital Accreditation specifies a "turn-around" time on document production, in order to meet their requirement for quality control. The medical transcriptionist position, therefore, is one that is vital to the day-to-day processing of patient information.

CHAPTER SUMMARY

Word processing is one of the most frequently used computer applications. Many software manufacturers produce word processing software. However, all word processors allow for basic functions to be performed. These basic functions include formatting, editing, printing, saving, and retrieving.

Other features may vary among the various word processing software packages available. Many allow for specialized features including merge and macro operations, math features, and viewing more than one document on the screen at the same time.

Documentation is available when word processing software is purchased. It aids the end-user in determining how to perform specific operations. Word processing may seem difficult to learn at first, but users generally find word processing to be an extremely effective productivity tool.

TERMINOLOGY AND REVIEW EXERCISES

Essential Vocabulary

word wrap
function keys
caps lock
toggle key
control key
alternate key

Essential Vocabulary *(continued)*

num lock
scroll lock
directional tab key
PrtSc
functions
features
formatting
editing
printing
retrieving
typeover mode
insert mode
default setting
block operations
move command
copy command
on-screen formatting
pagination
headers and footers
justification
widows and orphans
status line
hard and soft returns
scrolling
hyphenation
hard and soft hyphen
math feature
multicolumn output
merge operation
macros
windows
spell check and thesaurus
backup file
documentation
Desktop Publishing
user-friendly
menu driven
command driven

True/False

1. The insert mode allows the end user to type directly over previously written text.
2. A copy command allows a copy to be made of text, leaving the original text in its place while copying that text onto another location.
3. A move command is sometimes referred to as a "cut and paste" operation.
4. Hard and soft page breaks, in part, determine where the text will end on the page.
5. Grammar checkers are considered a specialized feature of most word processing packages marketed today.
6. A thesaurus will automatically identify a word or words in a document that have been overly used within the document.
7. A document file is a stored file of textual material.
8. An example of a footer might be the words "Chapter Five" listed at the bottom of every other page within the document.
9. Advanced word processing applications include printing text, merging, and document assembly.
10. The ESC key is only used to cancel a command that has not yet been executed.

Fill in the Blanks

1. Five essential word processing functions include ________________, ________________, ________________, ________________, and ________________.

2. Grammar and spell checkers are not be used as a replacement for ______________________________.
3. A ____________________ is a series of saved keystrokes.
4. ______________________ ______________________ operations are useful in the production of form letters that can be individualized so that correct information is placed in the proper location in each document.
5. The move command allows the end user to __________________ a portion of text and move it to a new location within the text or within another document.
6. A ________________________ identifies a document by some type of textual or numeric information listed at the top of a page.
7. ____ is a written description of exact procedures to use to perform the functions or features of a word processing software package.
8. The ________________ and ____________________ keys aid the user in performing editing functions.
9. ________ ______________ ______________ controls line formatting by deciding when the end of the line should occur; this process take place automatically.
10. The CAPS LOCK is a __________________ ____________; the function that CAPS LOCK performs is either on or off.

Review Questions

1. Describe the difference between the two modes of operation: insert and typeover.
2. Discuss functions and features of a word processing package.
3. Define widows and orphans.
4. Describe the difference between hard and soft hyphens.
5. Identify the errors in the following sentences. Are there any errors that a spell check would not find?
   a. Its a wonderful day.
   b. The patient brought their children with them for the office visit.
   c. Where have you left you stetheoscope?
   d. If things were differnt, what would you want to do?
   e. Mr. Dobsonfield's wife looks just like Mr. Dobsonfeld.

Chapter 5

Spreadsheets

Chapter Outline

OBJECTIVES

1. Define a spreadsheet.
2. Discuss the differences between the three modes of operation in a spreadsheet.
3. Identify the four types of cell entries and describe the differences between them.
4. Define a range. Describe the steps involved in setting a range or a global setting?
5. Define precedence and describe how it affects spreadsheet calculations.
6. Discuss the various formatting features normally available for use within a spreadsheet.
7. Discuss the difference between the move and copy commands within a spreadsheet.
8. Describe the difference between relative and absolute values.
9. Identify the rules for designing spreadsheets. Discuss why each of these rules is important.

While word processing programs may have played a vital role in office automation, electronic spreadsheets, the "number crunchers" have revolutionized business management. Electronic spreadsheets enable individuals to analyze data in new ways and at incredible speeds.

Electronic spreadsheets are software programs that allow for electronic calculations to be performed on designated rows and columns of numerical data. The first electronic spreadsheet, VisiCalc, was produced in 1979. Since that time, many spreadsheet software packages have been introduced. Lotus 1-2-3, produced by Lotus Development Corporation, marked an explosive interest in spreadsheet marketing and development. Now spreadsheets have increased their power in both the sophisticated graphics production and the number of business functions they perform. QuatroPro, produced by Borland International, is another well-known spreadsheet available today.

ESSENTIAL SPREADSHEET TERMINOLOGY

All spreadsheets, independent of manufacturer, possess certain similar characteristics, structures, and capabilities. A spreadsheet consists of a **worksheet**, made of empty **rows** and **columns**. The number of available rows and columns will vary by different spreadsheet packages. This factor will determine, in part, the power of the software; the higher the number of rows and columns, the more powerful the spreadsheet may be.

Cells and Cell Location

Each cell within a spreadsheet is unique. Each intersection of a row and column represents a physical location on the spreadsheet termed a **cell**. Columns are alphabetical, while rows are numbered. The identifying number and letter associated with the cell is termed a **cell location**. The number and character together are referred to as a cell's **coordinates**. The term the **cell address** also refers to the unique location of the cell within the worksheet.

When the number of rows and number of columns are multiplied together, the resulting product will equal the total number of available cells within the spreadsheet software package. Each of these available cells may be used to analyze data, by performing mathematical calculations on the numeric entries located within the cell, Figure 5–1.

Labels, Values, Formulas, and Special Functions

Each cell has the capacity to be filled with particular types of data. These **cell entries**, or data types, are: labels, values, formulas, and special functions.

Labels are cell entries upon which no mathematical operations will occur. The entries can be alphabetic, numeric, or special characters. Examples of labels might include a sales location, such as BOSTON, or a model number, such as AG16752.

Values are cell entries upon which mathematical operations can occur; values are, simply, numeric data. Values may be added to other values, subtracted, multiplied, or divided.

Labels may be numeric, such as in an identifying product number, consisting of only numeric characters. For example, a product number designated 67543 might reflect an automobile part on a warehouse inventory sheet. This number would be considered only a label so it would not be used in any mathematical operations.

Formulas may also be entered into cells. Formulas within a cell will direct mathematical operations to occur on entries made in other cells. The formula A1+B2+C2 entered into cell address, D2, for example, will result in the calculation of sum of the three numeric values located in each of the designated cell locations, A1, B2, and C2. The resulting

TAKE A MOMENT

	A	B	C	D	E	F	G
❑ 1							
❑ 2							
❑ 3							

How many rows are available in the above worksheet?

How many columns?

How many cells are available?

Figure 5-1

value or sum will be entered into the cell located at the intersection of the row 2 and the column D of the spreadsheet. This cell is, of course, identified by its cell coordinates (D and 2) and is given the unique cell location D2. Formulas are expressed by using the following symbols: + for addition, – for subtraction, * for multiplication, ^ for exponentiation, and a / for division.

Special functions may also be cell entries. Special functions allow for operations to occur on a single cell or a combination of cells. Typical special functions include averaging, adding, calculating square roots, and locating maximum values. Available special functions can vary from simple operations, such as AVG (average) or SUM (add together) to more complex statistical or financial operations.

Argument and Range

A **range** or **argument** in a spreadsheet is a designated group of cells. A range of cells may be any combination of adjacent cells. For example, cells at locations C1, C2, C3, D1, D2, and D3 may be combined to form a range. A range is established by entering in the cell location of the upper left cell to be included in the range. In this case, that cell location would be C1. Next the range is marked with a **delimiter**. The delimiter may vary but with most spreadsheet software it is either a period or a combination of periods. The delimiter marks the cell address as the beginning of a range. The final cell address of the range is then added. In this particular example, the cell address is D3, the bottom right hand cell location to be included in the range. Ranges are generally designated by the use of parentheses. The above range would be typed (C1..D3).

It is important to recognize that this range (C1..D3) will include all cell locations with values entered into the spreadsheet between the cell locations C1 and D3. If a value has been mistakenly entered into the cell C4, for example, that value would be used in all subsequent calculations. Ranges and arguments are error prone and must be checked and verified during each step of the spreadsheet development phase.

Precedence

Mathematical operations are performed in a predetermined order. **Precedence** is the term that designates the rules of order for mathematical operations. First, operations occur from the left to the right. Multiplication and division occurs before addition and subtraction. Exponential operations will occur first, before either addition and subtraction or multiplication and division. Parentheses will take precedence over other operations, but within parentheses, operations will proceed from left to right. Spreadsheet software will follow these basic rules of precedence. In order for spreadsheet formulas to function effectively, these rules must be observed when creating or designing a spreadsheet utilizing formulas.

Relatives and Absolutes

A cell location within a formula may be either relative or absolute. An **absolute cell address** contains a value or formula that will not change regardless of its position within the spreadsheet. Absolutes remain constant within a worksheet.

When a cell address is **relative**, the formula of the cell will change depending on its position within the worksheet. Most cell addresses need to be relative and reflect the appropriate changes based upon their location within the spreadsheet.

MODES OF OPERATION

Many spreadsheets are menu driven. Menus are choices shown on the screen in order to give the end user or computer operator a selection of available options. In order to enter the **command mode**, where choices can be made from the menu, depending upon which spreadsheet package being used, it may be necessary to strike the (/) slash key or another designated key. Most spreadsheets use the slash to enter the command mode, Figure 5–2.

```
A1:                                   MENU
Worksheet, Range, Copy, Move, File, Print
```

Figure 5–2 Sample control panel

The top three lines shown on the monitor in Lotus 1-2-3 are called a **control panel**. The control panel is roughly equivalent to a status line, giving the computer operator the basic information about the worksheet. The panel shown in Figure 5–2 tells the user the following information. In the upper right hand corner, the current mode of operation is listed. This notation is referred to as the **mode indicator**. In Lotus, the designation, MENU, represents the command mode. The command mode allows the user to input commands from the menu or to input other commands using the function keys. The cell coordinates, A and 1, listed in the second row locate the current cell.

Ready Mode

The **ready mode** is the mode of operation that accepts data entry into a particular cell. Movement from one cell to another can take place in this READY mode by moving the directional arrow keys. This mode may sometimes be called the entry mode. Once a location has been chosen, data entry can take place. Once entry of data into a cell has begun, generally another mode of operation may not be entered until that cell entry is completed.

Edit Mode

In order to make changes in a cell entry once an entry has been completed and entered into the spreadsheet, the ready or the edit mode must be used. The **edit mode**, as the name implies, allows the end user to make changes in a cell that already holds data. Some spreadsheets will automatically switch to an edit mode if an identifiable error has been made. When entering a formula, for example, if the operator does not key in the formula in the correct format, then the spreadsheet software returns to the edit mode at that cell location. The computer operator then has the opportunity to make the necessary correction. However, many errors may not be located by the software. For example, if the value of 100 should have been entered into the cell location, B3, and was accidentally entered into the cell location, C3, then the software may not "catch" the problem.

FORMATTING FEATURES

Spreadsheets allow for various formats to be used. These features enhance the spreadsheet in various ways and may vary from package to package, although many are now considered standard.

Numeric Formats

Spreadsheets can express values in a variety of ways. When dollar amounts are involved then often the formats of decimals and dollar signs are used. Scientific applications may call for the exponential expression of values. Exponential expression is considered a formatting feature. Numbers can be expressed with floating decimal places, or they can be rounded off at a predetermined number of decimal points. Values can also be expressed as percents, allowing for even another numeric format.

Column Formats

Columns within a worksheet can be formatted to specification. Features involved in columnar formatting include setting widths for each column, setting right or left justifications, or setting decimal alignments.

Both numeric and columnar formats may be set globally or by default. Default settings, again, are those initial settings determined by the manufacturer. These default settings may be changed within the spreadsheet by using the appropriate keystrokes to initiate the desired command. Settings may be changed for a single cell, a range of cells, or **globally**. Global changes mean changes which apply to every cell within the worksheet.

FUNCTION KEYS

The function key F1..F10 or F12 will perform particular commands commonly used within the spreadsheet format.

Often the function key, F1, will bring up the HELP screen. The Help Screen option can be used to refresh the user's memory about certain spreadsheet features. A common complaint from novice users is: "The HELP screen is really No HELP at all." Admittedly, it takes practice and patience to decipher how different packages organize their HELP function. However, it is definitely worth a user's time and effort to work with this function.

Being able to demonstrate competence in using HELP screens and documentation is one of the characteristics of an experienced user. The experienced user can generally work his own way out of a problem, even if the user doesn't know all the right answers to begin with.

Other function keys may be used to set formats or to move the **pointer** around the spreadsheet. The pointer in a spreadsheet will highlight the cell at the location of the cursor, or the location of the two cell coordinates. Usually function keys control **move** and/or **copy** operations in a spreadsheet. Move relocates a portion of the spreadsheet while copy makes an exact duplicate of a designated portion of the spreadsheet.

ADVANCED FEATURES OF SPREADSHEETS

Macros

Macros are available for use in spreadsheets. They are, as in word processing, a series of saved keystrokes. These keystrokes are used as a time-saving device when the same keystrokes are keyed in frequently by the user. The keystrokes used to make up a macro may be either simple characters or they may be characters in combination with a group of commands. Basically when a macro is implemented, the saved keystrokes are retrieved from their file and repeated within the new application.

Templates

Templates are a useful tool for designing and saving forms that may be reused over and over again. The spreadsheet worksheet is designed and developed without any of the variable numeric entries for the cells. Values that will change with each use of the form are left off the template. Labels, formulas, and special functions, as well as constant numeric values can all be entered into the template worksheet, leaving only the variable numeric values empty. Once the template is completed, it can be saved and retrieved for repeated use.

Windows

Windows are now available for use in some spreadsheet software packages. Computer operators can use window technology to view more than one spreadsheet or more than one section of a spreadsheet at the same time. Windows provide the user with the capability of making visual comparisons on the screen without printing a hard copy.

RULES FOR DESIGNING AND CONSTRUCTING SPREADSHEETS

The old computer adage "Garbage In, Garbage Out (GIGO)" certainly applies most aptly to designing and developing spreadsheets. If the values and formulas used to calculate information in the spreadsheet are inaccurate, then, of course, that information will be faulty. Countless examples of the "Garbage In, Garbage Out" phenomenon have caused innumerable problems for the organizations that relied on faulty information resulting from poorly designed spreadsheets. Generally, the problems that result from poor spreadsheet construction result in financial repercussions in some manner or another. Following some basic guidelines for the production of effective spreadsheets can alleviate these problems.

1. **Use a clear title.** The importance of a clear title cannot be overly stressed. A spreadsheet title needs to be a concise description of what the spreadsheet contains. The title needs to include all relevant information answering, if necessary, the basic questions of who, what, when, and where. For example, look at the sample spreadsheet title below.

   Average per Hospital Unit

   We know that the title refers to hospital units and that the numeric information found in the title is an average. The information, however, does not convey meaningful or useful figures. Questions concerning the data remain unanswered. Average what? Is it the average number of patients, or the average number of employees, or does it represent the average number of a particular type of equipment available? A more informative title might be one that includes a more complete description of what the "average" represents. In the sample spreadsheet title, no information is conveyed regarding when or what time frame these averages represent. Are these averages daily, monthly, or yearly composites of data?
2. **State the purpose of the spreadsheet.** The purpose of the information within the spreadsheet needs to be clearly defined. Purpose statements may be included in the title, if appropriate, or may be included in textual information provided with the spreadsheet. If attempting comparisons of employee absenteeism by hospital unit, then the spreadsheet title also needs to impart that knowledge.

An appropriate title for that type of spreadsheet might be: Comparison of Average Days Absence for Nursing Staff per Hospital Unit: March 1991. Clearly, the title must describe the type of data that is to be utilized in the worksheet and the type of information that will result.

3. **Use cell protection when needed.** If a spreadsheet is being developed as a template to be used repeatedly, then cells that have been developed containing the formulas for the template need to be protected from modification. Sometimes cell protection is available to the end user through the use of passwords, allowing access to the template where the formulas are entered only if the user knows the correct access code. Passwords are considered a computer security measure.
4. **Verify cell entries.** Proofreading and verifying correct cell entries should be considered an important aspect of creating a spreadsheet. If cell entries contain errors either in values or formulas, then the resulting data will be corrupt, that is, invalid. Often an individual creating a spreadsheet may not recognize all errors within it. If the information is to be used as a basis for important decisions relying on accurate results then a wise course of action might be to have the spreadsheet entries and formulas verified by an individual other than the original creator.

   Regardless of who does the proofing of the spreadsheet, documentation should be attached, including the formulas used in determining the values that the cells within the worksheet represent. A hard copy of formula statements for a spreadsheet can be printed. This procedure should be considered standard for all spreadsheets that reflect vital information.
5. **Define all formula assumptions.** Formulas often contain a number of assumptions that may not be clear to an individual who is reading a spreadsheet. For that reason it is important to provide that information as a part of the spreadsheet. Scientific analysis of data may result in statistically significant results. For example, certain statistical assumptions are made when significance is established. Levels of confidence in reported findings may be expressed and these should be available to the reader. It is not enough to say that the results are significant, the underlying definition of "significance" needs to be expressed.

CHAPTER SUMMARY

Spreadsheets are another popular type of productivity software. They allow the user to perform arithmetic operations on rows and columns of figures. Calculations made with the use of this software are fast and reliable.

A spreadsheet cell, the point of intersection between a row and a column, can be designated as a label, a value, a formula, or a special function. Labels are descriptive only and are not used in mathematical calculation, whereas values are. Formulas express a mathematical operation to be performed on other cells within a spreadsheet. Special functions may be any number of mathematical operations that the speadsheet can perform on designated cells, including financial analysis and statistical measurement. The basic terminology applicable to the use of spreadsheets is covered within the chapter.

Spreadsheets are extremely useful in producing information that can be applied to business management. Many of the features that spreadsheets provide are developed with these applications in mind. Guidelines that aid the user in designing effective spreadsheets need to be followed in order to prevent major flaws in the information produced.

TERMINOLOGY AND REVIEW EXERCISES

Essential Vocabulary

electronic spreadsheet
worksheet
rows
columns
cell
cell location
cell coordinate
cell address
label
value
special function
range
argument
delimiter
precedence
absolute cell address
relative cell address
command mode
control panel
mode indicator
ready mode
edit mode
numeric format
columnar format
global formatting
pointer
macros
templates
windows
cell protection
formula assumptions

True/False

1. Precedence rules suggest that addition and subtraction always precede exponentiation.
2. Labels that are numeric may be included in arithmetic operations.
3. Relative numbers never change their values when moved to a new location within a spreadsheet.
4. Formulas that are entered into cells may be printed as a part of documentation for the contents of the spreadsheet.
5. Range and argument are synonymous terms referring to a designated group of cells.
6. Spreadsheet commands "move" and "copy" both make a copy of a section of the spreadsheet, while the "move" command leaves one copy in its original place.
7. A control panel is that section of the spreadsheet that allows the end user to enter formulas.
8. Modes of operation include ready, edit, and entry.
9. Numeric formats can include decimal points and scientific notation.
10. A global format refers to the fact that every cell within a spreadsheet will possess that same format.

Fill in the Blanks

1. The ____________ mode in a spreadsheet allows the end user to make changes in a cell that already holds data.
2. ____________________ ____________________ includes setting widths for a column, setting right or left justifications, or setting decimal alignments.
3. ______________________ are a series of saved keystrokes that can be a time-saving device for lengthy keystroke sequences used frequently.
4. ____________________ are a useful tool for saving formats that will be used over again.
5. ____________________ ________________________ blocks entry of new data or changes of any data that have previously been entered and saved.
6. ____________________ ______________________ should be accomplished for every new spreadsheet design and could result in helping the spreadsheet user prevent costly errors.
7. The ____________ ______ __________ of a cell make up its address or identifies its location.
8. Rows are marked with ________________________ in a spreadsheet while columns are marked with ________________.
9. ____________________________ are numeric cell entries that may be used in mathematical operations.
10. ________________________ within a spreadsheet will direct mathematical operations to occur and the value of the operation to be entered into the appropriate cell.

Review Questions

1. List and discuss the guidelines for constructing spreadsheets.
2. Discuss the benefits of cell protection.
3. Discuss the importance of cell verification.
4. Define and distinguish between labels, values, formulas, and special functions.
5. Distinguish between relative and absolute values.

Chapter 6

Database Software and Information Management

Chapter Outline

OBJECTIVES

1. Define a data base.
2. Identify the structures within a data base.
3. Distinguish between the various data entry operations as applied to database systems.
4. Identify and discuss sorting and indexing within a data base.
5. Identify and discuss the types of database organization.
6. Discuss information systems development procedures.
7. Describe various types of information systems and their typical applications.

Another powerful methodology for using the computer to process raw data and to provide information is that of database management. Database software provides a systematic information management tool that allows for the conversion of data into useful, meaningful information. Recall that data are the raw facts that have been collected. Once these raw facts have been processed by a computer system, information becomes available for use. Data can be organized in data structures, moving from simple data structures to the most complex, the data base itself. This chapter examines data within the data hierarchy, frequently used data entry operations employed in database software, and the various types of database organization used in information systems.

DATABASE ESSENTIALS

Fields

Fields are the basic data categories within the data base. Fields can be either numeric, alphanumeric, logical, or memo. (Each of these fields are composed of bits and bytes.) Fields are designated as columns in a database file.

Alphanumeric fields may contain virtually any character on the computer keyboard. These fields may consist of letters, numbers, and special characters, symbols, or punctuation such as *,#,@ and ^. For example, a person's social security number would be considered an alphanumeric field because it contains both numeric and special characters, the numbers and the dash characters that separate them. Another example of an alphanumeric field would be a person's address, because it contains both numbers and letters. Alphanumeric fields are not used in calculations and may be referred to also as **character fields**.

Numeric fields, as the name implies, consists of a number or numbers (0,1,2, . . . 9), and may also include the special characters of a period, a decimal point, or a hyphen (constituting a negative number). If arithmetic operations are to be performed on the data fields, then those fields must be numeric. However, numeric fields may also be used as labels with no arithmetic value. For example a product code label, 643579, is numeric because it consists of a combination of numbers. Even though it is composed of numbers, it is descriptive in intent. This product code number would never be used in addition or subtraction with another product code number or another numeric value.

Logical fields consist of either one of two possible values such as True or False, Yes or No, or Male or Female. An example of this type of field might be used on a employee's information file indicating in response to the category "employed over 5 years," with the response being either Yes or No.

Memo fields are fields that can be used to add data that may be unique to a particular record. Memo fields are usually used as a documentation device, providing some type of reference material for the computer operator.

Field length, the maximum number of characters available within a field, is generally limited by the software manufacturer. Other variations may include the maximum number of possible fields and the maximum number of records. It is extremely important to be aware of these variations before making purchasing decisions about prepackaged database management software.

Records

Related fields are grouped together in a **record**. The fields within a record are always organized in the same order. The particular order is referred to as the **record structure** and does not change from one record to another. If a logical field for Male and Female is found in the fourth field in the first record, then that same logical field will also be located in the fourth field in other records within the same file.

Records within a particular file will always have the same number of fields. The rows of the database file are designated as the records. Each record will be marked in some way that allows for the recognition of its location within the file. This **record location** within the file is called the record number or **record address**.

Files

Files are a collection of related records. Examples of database files are numerous.

A wholesale service business might maintain a file containing information on all the businesses retained as customers. This particular type of file would contain records, probably one record per customer, with fields relating to the name of the company, its address, the business's phone number, the type of business it is, and the legal owner of the business. This same wholesale business may maintain another completely different database file containing information on all the employees of the company. The employee database file would, of course, contain records, one per employee, that provide fields of information related to that employee.

The Data Base

A **data base** is the highest level of organization within the **data hierarchy**. The data hierarchy ranks data from its most simple form, the bit, to its most complex, the database itself. The term data base refers to the collection of information that represents all fields, records, and files. **Database software** or database management software is a prepackaged software that aids the user in creating and using a data base. This includes adding and deleting records within the data base, extracting information from existing records within the data base, and allowing for the creation of new files from the existing records.

DATA ENTRY OPERATIONS

All data bases require the completion of data entry operations. Three basic data entry operations may occur within the database system: additions, deletions, and modifications. These data entry operations constitute what is generally referred to as **file updating** or **file maintenance**. These operations must occur on a regular basis if the information within the data base is to be kept current.

Additions and Deletions

When a new patient enters a hospital that stores patient information in a database system, that patient's record must be added to the information system. This process will require the file maintenance data entry operation of **addition**. All required fields of information must be collected and then entered into the system. Depending upon the particular software system being used, additions of this type may be **appended** (added the record to the end of the file, or **inserted**, (added between two existing records). Hospital admissions personnel may make additions to the information system directly or may create a **source document** to be processed by data entry personnel. At times the source document, the hard copy from where the data originated, may be required for backup in case of data loss. By storing source documents, organizations protect themselves from the possibility of important or essential data becoming irretrievable.

Because the data contained in information fields within the records of a database are important, deletions must always be approached with caution. **Deletions** of pertinent information can be time-consuming to repair. Sometimes reconstruction is possible but frequently it is lost and cannot be retrieved. Because data loss may occur, efforts must be directed towards proper use of this data entry operation. The rule is to double check *always* when deleting material. Make sure that the record being deleted is the correct one before actually making the deletion.

Some software systems provide a two step procedure which aids recovery if deletion occurs accidently. First, the record is **logically deleted**, and marked accordingly. The logical deletion keeps that particular record out of current processing tasks but does not physically delete it. It is possible to add the record back into the system at this point by using an **undelete** procedure. The undelete procedure removes the logically deleted record and returns it to its original place within the file. Of course, after complete **physical deletion**, the record is no longer part of the system and must be readded if needed.

Modification and Verification

Changes to an existing record may be made by the process of editing. Your database software system will have a specific command procedure for you to follow in order to enter an edit mode. This procedure (called **data modification**) will require locating and retrieving the record in which changes must be made, then keying in the new data (such as a new address or phone) over the existing entry.

The importance of correct data entry cannot be overemphasized. Once all updating has been completed, it is best to go back and proofread updates one final time. This process of **data verification** is an ongoing task that should not be overlooked.

TYPICAL DATABASE OPERATIONS

While calculations are the "meat and potatoes" of the daily spreadsheet user's diet, database users generally feast on sorts and indexes. Let's examine what these terms mean and how they can add to the productive functioning of an organization.

Sorting

Recall that **sorting** is a data processing operation; sorting arranges information in a particular order or defined sequence. Typically sorts include:

- **ascending numeric sorts**, starting with the smallest number and proceeding through to the largest numeric value: 1,2,3 . . . 7,8,9,0.
- **ascending alphabetic sorts**, starting with the first letter of the alphabet and proceeding through until the last letter in the sequence is covered: A,B,C, . . . W,X,Y,Z.
- **descending numeric sorts**, starting with the largest numeric value and proceeding through to the smallest: 15436,15420 . . . . 15000.
- and **descending alphabetic sorts**, starting with the last possible letter of the alphabet and returning to the very first letter: Z,T,Q,B . . . A.

Sorts may be accomplished by establishing more than one field by which to sort the records within a data base. Using more than one field in a sort operation is referred to as a **multiple sort**.

When more than one sort field has been established, it is necessary to identify which field is to be sorted first. This field is identified as the **primary sort key**. Sorting with a primary sort key can also be referred to as a **major sort**. The second field within the sort sequence would be identified as a **secondary sort key**, or referred to as a **minor sort**. Any sorts following the secondary sort will also be minor sorts. The number of available **key fields** (fields that may be utilized by any one sort procedure) will vary among software package manufacturers.

Figure 6–1 is a list of new employees for a teaching hospital. Each individual's data has been entered into a database file.

RECORD	LASTNAME	FIRSTNAME	PH.D.	DPT.NO.*	TITLE
1	DAVIDSON	GEORGE	Y	006	PROFESSOR
2	DAVIDSON	ANNE	N	003	LECTURER
3	WILSON	BEN	Y	003	PROFESSOR
4	WINTER	PAULA	Y	006	PROFESSOR
5	MARTINEZ	HENRY	Y	002	LECTURER
6	JOHNSON	MARIE	Y	006	ASST.PROFESSOR

Figure 6–1 Sample database file

For each employee certain information has been collected and entered into the fields. For sake of illustration, the fields have been limited. The collection of all records is the database file. Note the difference between the rows and columns. The rows make up the records, and the columns contain the fields. Each record will have the same number of fields associated with it . . . in this case, six.

Sorting information could occur on one of several of the fields. A single ascending alphabetic sort might be used with the key field designated, LAST NAME. However, since some employees have the same last name, a multiple ascending alphabetic sort on the key fields LAST NAME and FIRST NAME might be a more productive alternative. For

*DPT.NO. refers to department number

particularly large organizations with thousands of employees, sorts might be required using more key fields, including middle initials or addresses.

A numeric sort might be utilized ranking all employees on the basis of their department number. In this case, a sort would serve to group all employees of the same department together. Such information might be valuable to have when appropriations are being made for new staff.

Sorts can occur on logical fields also. Sorts employing the logical fields as one key field (of at least two) may also be called **conditional sorts**. An example of a conditional sort on the above file would be sort all teachers having Ph.D.s by department in ascending alphabetic order.

Indexing Files

As with sorts, indexes may be based on one or more data fields. **Indexing** creates a file based upon the key fields it utilizes, leaving the original intact. A **pointer** is set up as a field within the indexed file in order to establish and maintain the sequence of records as they existed in the original file. Figure 6–2 will clarify how an indexing procedure occurs.

The original file is an alphabetic list of patients with account balances. The file has five fields. The original record number is considered a field as is the last name, zip code, and account balance. Again, fields are limited for clarity. In an actual patient file, you would find more fields, including first name, address, account number, etc., Figure 6–2.

ORIGINAL FILE RECORD	LASTNAME	ZIP CODE	BALANCE	POINTER
1	ANDREWS	78209	3276.47	2
2	DONOVAN	07642	925.76	3
3	JENSON	53240	4720.00	4
4	KNOX	98437	840.90	5
5	PHILLIPS	24368	1456.58	EOF

Figure 6–2 Patient balance file

Fields include both the record number and the pointer number in the original file. The letters **EOF** mark the end of the file, meaning that there are no more records past record number 5. The pointer number will give the original position of the record even after it has been indexed.

To create an indexed file that ranks the patient's zip code in ascending order the proper fields to be sorted would be identified. Notice how after the sort has been accomplished, the record numbers and the pointer fields change position. The original file is maintained in proper sequence through the pointer field, Figure 6–3. Another example of an indexed file is one that ranks all records by the descending account balance, Figure 6–4.

INDEXED ORIGINAL FILE SORTED BY ZIP CODE				
RECORD	LASTNAME	ZIP CODE	BALANCE	POINTER
1	DONOVAN	07642	925.76	3
2	PHILLIPS	24368	1456.58	EOF
3	JENSON	53240	4720.00	4
4	ANDREWS	78209	3276.47	2
5	KNOX	98437	840.90	5

Figure 6–3 Patient balance file indexed by zip code

INDEXED FILE SORTED BY DESCENDING BALANCE				
RECORD	LASTNAME	ZIP CODE	BALANCE	POINTER
1	JENSON	53240	4720.00	4
2	ANDREWS	78209	3276.47	2
3	PHILLIPS	24368	1456.58	EOF
4	DONOVAN	07642	925.76	3
5	KNOX	98437	840.90	5

Figure 6–4 Patient balance file indexed by descending account balance

TYPES OF DATABASE REPORTS

Summary Reports

Summary reports involve counting and totaling different fields within the file records. Some examples:

- all patient accounts could be counted and totaled for a summary total of all active accounts
- one summary might count and total all patients who have not been seen in the last year
- another report counts all employees who have a minimum annual starting salary of $25,000 a year

This last report would involve simple counts of the employees with that salary or above and give a total. Generally, summary operations involve counting, subtotals, and totals.

Summary reports can be useful to both management and production personnel. Business examples of summary reports might involve total sales figures for a month sorted by a field that designates individual sales representatives. The sales representatives can see quickly whether they are meeting sales objectives. Management can make the necessary adjustments to support sales representatives through appropriate means. The types of summary reports can be as varied as the types of organizations that exist in the marketplace today.

The type of information sought and the reliability of the results are determined by the needs of the organization and the effective design of the summary report. Further examples include:

- A summary report of total number of employees sorted by individual departments. This could give top level management the necessary budgetary projections for personnel in the coming years.
- A summary report of new accounts sorted by branch office. This could give a home office new insight into effective sales procedures.
- Branch offices exceeding sales quotas consistently might be studied more closely to learn effective sales strategies that could be used throughout the company's various locations.

Exception Reports

Database software systems allow for the development of exception reports: (reports that choose or select only those records within a file that show some unique characteristic). For a hospital, an example of an exception report might include the number of nosocomial infections occurring, sorted by individual hospital units. This information allows for appropriate followup of these patients. It also aids in tracking the cause of the infections if they are occurring repeatedly in the same location.

Accounting departments within hospitals or group practices might utilize another type of exception report. For example, the exception report could list patient account records that are overdue more than 120 days. A decision could be reached on each of these accounts as to the appropriate means for collection of the past due amount.

The purpose of the exception report is to earmark records that may require particular attention by the employees of an organization. Businesses might want to identify gross sales above a certain amount by individual sales representatives. Such a report might result in recognition for the outstanding employee in some way—perhaps by both the sales manager (contributing a friendly handshake and comment), and the payroll department (adding a bonus to the individual's regular paycheck).

Detail Reports

These reports provide listings of every record within a file. Continuing with our previous example, a file maintaining sales representatives and the amount of their monthly sales might make up a detail report. Sales managers might use this listing to oversee the total sales operations. A detail report of this type might be prepared utilizing an ascending alphabetical sort so that each sales representative's name would be listed alphabetically along with the amount of sales made for that month. The report might be summarized by adding the total sales for each representative giving subtotal categories and finally reporting a total sales figure for the entire operation for that month.

Preparing Reports. Reports are generally produced by printing a hard copy for circulation to the appropriate personnel. Certain information needs to be included in any formal report. The report should have an appropriate title. Additionally:

- Fields or columns need to be defined.
- Use of any abbreviations within the fields should be clarified.
- Summary fields must also be defined so that the report will appear in a clear and concise manner, consistent with a professional document.

Since reports are prepared periodically, as they are required, the operating procedure for preparing the report needs to be maintained for future reference. This documentation should outline the format for the report, including line spacings, tab settings, and any other unusual features. Fields to be calculated should be specified along with the directions for completing any calculations that need to be performed. The name of the original designer of the report might be a useful addition to the documentation for the report in case any questions arise pertaining to its production. Documentation of this type provides a backup for individuals who need to know what is expected in preparing these periodic reports. New employees will find these backups extremely practical when confronting the challenges of productivity in a new position.

DATABASE ORGANIZATION AND SYSTEMS DEVELOPMENT

Three commonly used database concepts that reflect the organization or method by which data is stored within the database are relational, network, and hierarchical.

Relational Data bases

Relational database software is particularly popular for use on microcomputers since the volume of data involved in the database is relatively small. Simply, in a relational database, relationships between individual records exist. In this type of database a field may be unique to a particular record and is identified as the key field. Social security numbers and patient identification numbers are good examples of frequently used key fields. All other fields within the record are descriptive and these fields are called **attributes**. In all records the fields are consistent. For example, the LASTNAME field in the file has ten spaces reserved for that field. The LASTNAME field will always contain 10 spaces whether the field contains the name JONES or GOLDSMITH. If the last name to be entered within a field contains more than the allowed 10 characters, the last characters will be automatically left off.

Hierarchical Data bases

A **hierarchical** relationship is established among the records in what is commonly referred to as a tree structure which resembles an organizational chart. The top level record is called the parent record and is related in some manner to each of the lower level records, called child records. This type of organization for a data base is generally restricted to large computer systems.

Network Data Bases

The organization of the **network data base** is the most complex. Its use is also restricted to larger computer systems. In a network structure records can be related among several different files.

PROGRAMMING PREPACKAGED DATABASE SYSTEMS

Each organization is unique even though most organizations maintain similar types of information, such as financial or accounting records, inventory records, and personnel records. Organizations and the people in them decide what particular kinds of information they need and can use. Colleges need to maintain information on the courses they teach and the number of available classrooms and teachers. Hospitals need to maintain records on their patients and their unique needs.

In order for an organization to be effective, it must be responsive to the people it serves. In order to employ prepackaged database information systems to their optimal capacity, the ability to program a database to serve the individual and unique information needs of the organization is required. Prepackaged database software that allows an organization flexibility in database design is now available to meet these needs.

INFORMATION SYSTEMS

Data is entered into a computer system by computer operators. Various calculations, summaries, or categorizations take place through data processing occurring in the central processing unit of the computer system. The end result is the output, whether it resides on the screen, is saved to a disk or other storage medium, or is prepared as a hard copy of printed material. The output can be used by the computer operators themselves or can be used by others within the organization.

The information input and output, the computer system components, and the people who employ the processed data in various tasks—all these individual factors make up an **information system**. It is no small task to develop a working system that can integrate all of these factors successfully, merging sound principles of management with complex processing technology to produce vital information.

Categories of Information Systems

There are a number of categories of business functions that have utilized information systems to fulfill data processing requirements and produce the required information. Some of these categories are:

- Management information systems
- Marketing information systems
- Accounting information systems
- Financial analysis information systems
- Specialized information systems

These systems provide organizations with information in varying forms. From the descriptions below, the variety of applications utilizing information systems can be realized.

Management Information Systems. Management is categorized by the functions or activities it performs. Each of these managerial functions must be performed in even the smallest of organizations. Management functions or activities include planning, organizing, staffing, directing, and supervising.

ACTIVITIES/FUNCTIONS OF MANAGEMENT	LEVELS OF MANAGEMENT
Planning and policy making	Top level
Organization and staffing	Middle
Direction and supervision	Lower level

1. Generally lower level managers are directly involved in the supervision of employees and in overseeing daily operations.
2. Middle level managers make decisions on organizational problems and personnel issues related to organizational goals.
3. Top level managers are concerned with policy making and long range planning.

Effective management information systems support all aspects of managerial activities from top level to lower, from supplying information upon which policy decisions are reached at the top level of management, to lower level functions by supporting supervisory activities.

The computer system makes information available to individuals within an organization in a timely and efficient manner. This information, necessary and vital to effective day to day functioning, aids the individual members of the organization in goal orientation and goal achievement.

Marketing Information Systems. Customers come in all different shapes and sizes. They may buy clothes, other goods, or services for themselves or their families. These purchases may be cash or credit based. Kids are customers, too. They make choices on the games they play, the tennis shoes they wear, and the candy they want for a treat. Patients are also customers, selecting the hospitals and clinics they want to use or the kind of insurance they think is important. The examples are endless.

One fact is certain, however. When purchases are being made, data is being collected about the people involved in the purchase and about the type of purchase they are making. What do they purchase? What type of products? How many? What size or color? How much did the item cost?

Marketing information systems take the raw data about the particular purchases being made and create information that will be useful to an organization attempting to maintain its position in the marketplace. Information will be created that aids the marketing department in creating products that people will buy. This information will also be used to guide advertising promotions and pricing policies as well as shape inventories.

Accounting Information Systems. Accounting business functions are an essential part of any organization. Funds for the cost of raw materials are necessary before manufacturing can take place and sales of manufactured products can occur. Cash reserves for meeting payroll must be available even for a nonprofit organization before organizational functions can proceed.

Accounting systems serve to monitor and oversee the cash flow of an organization. These systems streamline all the accounting functions of the organization, helping the organization to continue as a viable entity. Computerized accounting systems may cover all or part of an organization's accounting needs. Generally the functions they facilitate include accounts receivable and payable, payroll, sales invoicing and related record keeping, and inventory control.

Financial Analysis Information Systems. While the accounting functions are necessary for day to day operations, decision making often requires more complex analysis of an organization's information. Financial analysis can provide a measurement of an organization's viability through income and balance sheet statements. Analysis also provides information that predicts, based upon past performance, what can be expected to happen in the future. This type of analysis is referred to as financial forecasting.

Corporations that sell stock to the public are often analyzed financially. This type of financial analysis may result in a financial rating (a measurement that predicts the organization's ability to perform well).

Financial analysis can be used internally by an organization to decide on allocation of resources. A hospital administrator, for example, may use financial analysis to predict the amount of available funds (revenues, etc.); on the basis of these figures funds can be allocated to the various departments according to the department's financial requirements and the hospital's ability to meet them.

Past accounting statements of an organization, large or small, provide the input or raw data for financial analysis. In a large organization, information might be shared between two different departments: accounting and finance. The accounting department supplies the top level management with information and the finance department with raw data. Finance, after completing their own analysis, would also report findings to the top level managers.

Specialized Information Systems. Specialized systems have been developed to meet unique organizational needs. Information systems have been developed for such diverse industries as automobile retail sales operations, real estate brokerages, banking, and, of course, medical facilities. The information systems developed particularly for medical facilities will be covered in detail in the next chapters.

FACTORS IN DESIGNING OR SELECTING INFORMATION SYSTEMS

Information systems can be designed to meet specific organizational requirements or they can be selected from a variety of prepackaged systems to meet organizational needs. Several factors need to be considered in selecting or designing information systems.

- **The system life cycle.** The decision to consider implementing an information system leads to a number of steps that are generally referred to as the **system life cycle.**

The system life cycle consists of five phases: system assessment and analysis, system design, system development, system implementation, and system evaluation and maintenance.

Designing system requirements involves working through the phases of the system life cycle by following a series of guidelines needed for successful development of a working system. These guidelines generally are followed through the help of a **systems analyst**, a professional with specialized computer training that designs and implements computer systems. If an organization does not employ their own systems analyst, then they may be faced with contracting for the services of one.

- **The human factor.** Some information systems analysts define systems only in terms of input, processing, and output requirements. While these factors are worthy of careful and exhaustive study, they form an incomplete picture. The people who interact with the input and output operations are essential elements in any information system. Design requirements must include the human factor in any systems assessment, development, and implementation. This factor must be considered when deciding on additions of computer components and technology to an organization, particularly in health care organizations.

CHAPTER SUMMARY

Database management software can be an effective information management tool when integrated into an organization in an effective manner. Data within a data base is structured in a hierarchical fashion from the simplest to the most complex. The terms field, record, file, and data base represent these data structures.

Frequent operations when using database management software involve adding to and deleting data from the data base itself. Modification of existing data is also required. One essential operation is that of data verification (making certain that the data that is entered into the system is correct).

Database software systems are used to generate reports. These reports can be classified as summary reports, exception reports, and detail reports. Different levels of management use these reports as decision making tools.

Information systems that utilize database management software can be very complex. Many factors need to be considered before implementing a database system. Generally, for large organizations, a process referred to as the system life cycle may be required to effectively implement a new database system.

TERMINOLOGY AND REVIEW EXERCISES

Essential Vocabulary

fields
alphanumeric fields
character fields
numeric fields
logical fields
memo fields

field length
record
record structure
record location
record address
file
data base
data hierarchy
database software
file update
file maintenance
addition
append
insert
source document
deletion
logical deletion
physical deletion
undelete
data modification
data verification
sorting
ascending numeric sort
ascending alphabetic sort
descending alphabetic sort
descending numeric sort
multiple sort
primary sort key
major sort
secondary sort key
minor sort
key fields
indexing
conditional sorts
pointer
EOF
summary report
exception report
detail report
relational data base
attributes
hierarchical data base
network data base
information system
management information system
marketing information system
accounting information system
financial analysis information system
specialized information system
system life cycle
systems analyst

True/False

1. A data base is a collection of related files.
2. Alphanumeric fields contain only the letters of the alphabet and numbers.
3. Memo fields are created as a documentation device to reference unique facts about a record.
4. The record number will designate the location of the record within a database file.
5. The number of files within a data base can vary depending on the particular business applications needed by an organization.
6. File maintenance would not include appending, deleting, or inserting records within a file.
7. Deletions may be temporarily or permanently removed from a file.
8. Data verification requires proofreading and double checking all file updates.
9. If a primary sort key identifies the field, FIRST NAME, and sorts by ascending alphabetic sort, then the LAST NAME will be sorted alphabetically along with the FIRST NAME.
10. Indexing creates a completely new file with the records reorganized according to sort fields.

Fill in the Blanks

1. A ________________ ________________ uses a logical field as one key field.
2. A ________________ maintains the original record sequence in an indexed file.
3. ________________ ________________ contain listings of all records within a file.
4. ________________ ________________ earmark records that meet unique conditions.
5. ________________ ________________ involve counting and totaling fields within the records of a file.
6. ________________ ________________ structures provide a means for individual records to be linked through a unique field termed the ________________ ________________.
7. ________________ ________________ structures are the most complex database organization.
8. An ________________ ________________ consists of related factors of input, output, computer components, and the people who work with computer technology.
9. The system life cycle consists of several phases. These phases are accomplished through the professional assistance of a ________________ ________________.
10. A________________ ________________ ________________ ________________ may complete financial forecasting projections or help allocate financial resources.

Review Questions

1. Discuss the various information systems and the types of information they might provide.
2. List the phases of the system life cycle.
3. List and discuss the types of database reports that might typically be used within an organization.
4. Define the basic data entry operations used in a data base.
5. Discuss the major differences between sorting and indexing.

Chapter 7

Communications and Networking

Chapter Outline

OBJECTIVES

1. Define data communications channels.
2. Identify and define the types of data transmission.
3. Define and distinguish between synchronous and asynchronous transmission.
4. Identify the types of directional data flow.
5. Identify the three categories of bandwidth.
6. Identify common communication links.
7. Distinguish between communication service carriers and value added networks.
8. Identify hardware and software utilized in data communications.
9. Identify three network configurations.
10. Identify types of technology utilized in office automation.

DATA COMMUNICATIONS

Data communications refers to the transfer of data over a particular distance. **Data communications** can occur between computers and terminals within the same room or communications can occur over a greater distance, between a computer and a terminal within a building, a city, or even across thousands of miles.

Types of Transmission

Data transmission, the actual movement of data across communications lines, is often classified by how the basic data are transferred. These classifications include serial versus parallel transmission and asynchronous versus synchronous transmission. Simplex, half duplex, and full duplex transmission categorize directional flow of the transferring data. Each of these types of transmissions will be defined here.

Serial Transmission. One of the most common types of data transmission is known as **serial transmission**. Data communications occurs serially when data is transferred one bit at a time in a sequential fashion. For example, a byte of data 0100001 would be transferred 0, then 1, then 0 until the complete byte had been transmitted.

Parallel Transmission. In **parallel transmission** data is transferred by transmitting all bits in a byte at one time. Parallel transmission is faster than transmission occurring over serial lines and this is its major advantage. However, it is also more expensive so the increased cost needs to be justified by the need for speed in transmitting data and information.

Synchronous and Asynchronous Transmission. Data transmission is often categorized by how characters or bytes are moved. **Asynchronous transmission** refers to bytes being moved one at a time while **synchronous transmission** refers to a *group* of bytes being moved at a time.

Asynchronous transmission marks the passage of a byte of data with what is known as a start bit (marking the beginning), and a stop bit (marking the end of the data transmission). Data travels one byte at a time so if data loss occurs it will be minimal. Since data is transferred one byte at a time, data transmission is considerably slower than synchronous movement.

Synchronous transmission uses specialized timing devices between the terminals and computer for the purpose of monitoring the movement of data. Because data may be moved in large chunks at one time, this type of transmission is faster. However, if data loss occurs it may mean a large amount of work will have to be reentered into the system. This replication might be costly.

Simplex, Half-duplex and Full Duplex transmission. The direction of data flow may also be used to categorize transmission. These three categories are called simplex, half-duplex, and full duplex transmission.

Simplex transmission. In this type of transmission data is transferred in one direction only. Terminals connected to a computer with this type of transmission can either receive data or input data. This type of transmission is used less frequently than others.

Half-duplex transmission. Data with half-duplex transmission can travel in both directions, either to or from a terminal. However, data can only be moved in one direction at a time. One transmission must be complete before another can move across the line.

Full duplex transmission. With full duplex transmission data can move simultaneously in either direction. This type of transmission is the most commonly used.

Transmissions Speed

When data transmission channels or communication lines move data, the speed at which bits are transmitted is measured in bits per second (**bps**). The measurement may sometimes be called *line speed,* ie., the speed at which bits are transferred over a communications channel. In high speed networks, line speed may be measured in **Mbps** (million bits per second). A bps is the equivalent of a **baud**.

Bandwidth is a measurement that refers to the number of bits that may be carried over a communications line (type of cable) or other physical medium for transmitting data. There are three categories of bandwidth: narrowband, voiceband, and broadband.

Narrowband transmits at 45 to 300 bps. This line speed is the slowest of all bandwidth categories. An example of its application is telegraph transmission.

Voiceband transmission lines have a line speed range of 1800 to 9600 bps and are used in telephone or voice transmissions. This bandwidth is probably the most commonly used at the present time.

Broadband transmits at a line speed over 9600 bps and can reach speeds of 500,000 more bits per second. These types of transmission lines are used when high speed of transmission is required along with the transfer of large amounts of data and is currently the most expensive type of data transmission channel.

Types of Communications Lines

The most common types of communications links include telephone lines, coaxial cables, microwave transmission, satellites, and fiberoptics. Telephone lines are voiceband lines consisting of pairs of wires joined into a cable. Telephone lines can be used to transmit data, voices, or even images.

Coaxial lines are a broadband means of data transmission. These lines consist of bundles of wires enclosed in a durable shield, used to protect the lines from environmental hazards. Coaxial cables can be used over short or long distances; they transmit data faster than telephone lines, and can be used in an office environment or laid underground or undersea.

Microwaves are a type of broadband transmission that uses high frequency radiowaves which travel through space to transmit data along a route. **Satellites** are another type of broadband transmission. Data is beamed to a satellite that will reflect the data to another location. These satellites are orbiting in space around the earth receiving and transmitting signals.

Fiberoptics is a relatively new technology that allows for a means of transmitting data at high broadband speeds. The fiber optic cables transmit data using laser beams and allow for a greater amount of data to be transferred.

Communications Service Carriers

Communication lines may be privately or publicly owned and operated. They may be as simple as a connection between a printer and office computer or as complex as a satellite system. These lines are generally privately owned and operated. Most lines involved in long distance data communications are owned by companies which lease their services to the public. Common carriers offer data communications directly to the public. Examples include telephone and telegraph companies.

Value Added Networks (VANs)

Value added carriers such as **Telenet** and **Tymnet** offer specialized services to their customers but may not own their data transmission channels. Value added carriers group data into "packets" for transmission and may be cost effective for large data volumes.

Hardware and Software for Data Communications

Modems are hardware devices which convert digital signals to analog signals for transfer over communication lines or links (referred to as modulation). When modulation has been accomplished, demodulation, the reconversion to digital signals, occurs at the receiving location. This process also occurs through a modem. Hence the term, modem, has been shortened and stands for the modulation-demodulation process.

Several different types of modems are available. The **external direct-connect modem** is available as an add-on hardware component to a computer system. External modems can be transferred from one compatible system to another. **Internal direct-connect modems** are connected inside the computer housing. Modems, both external and internal, may be programmed to complete routine functions such as dialing automatically. Time delay features available on some modems allow for programming a data transfer to occur at another time, permitting users to transfer data during lower cost transfer periods.

Multiplexors are hardware that serve to concentrate messages from several small data communications lines for more efficient transfer through a transmission channel. Devices called remote concentrators may also fulfill this function within a communications network.

Control of the many functions necessary for data communications to occur within a large network may be accomplished through the use of a **front-end processor**. The processor relieves the main computer of these routine housekeeping duties, freeing the main computer or central processing unit for other processing tasks.

Data communications software is designed to regulate the data transmission functions in a number of ways. Some software allows for controlled communications between microcomputers and mainframes. When such communications occur, it is often necessary to provide mechanisms for access into particular files or databanks. Passwords to protect data from unauthorized use may be used. Other packages may be designed for communications among a group of microcomputers. The type of software required for a system will depend on the type of computers used, their locations, the amount of data transferred, protection requirements, and other factors.

DISTRIBUTED PROCESSING CONFIGURATIONS

Distributed processing refers to processing that takes place when two or more computers are linked with data communication lines. These systems of computers are often referred to as distributed processing networks and may be configured in a number of ways.

The **star configuration** consists of a host or main computer connected to one or more smaller computers. In the star system all communications between computers must pass through the host computer. A major disadvantage of a star configuration is that of downtime. If the host computer is not working, then no communications can occur.

The **ring configuration** has no host computer. Point to point contact occurs through the lines moving from one computer to the next. Breakdown in one computer in the ring configuration does not stop communications between the other computers since the data can be rerouted along the system. This operational reliability is one of the ring configuration's major advantages.

The **bus configuration** permits a computer to be connected anywhere within the system. This network system allows for reliable operations since it is not dependent upon a host computer. It differs from a ring configuration in that it does not have a circular arrangement. Bus networks are becoming the most widely used configuration.

Local area networks (LANs) are computers linked together by communications lines. LANs are generally located within close physical proximity to each other, within the same building or building complex. Local area networks can be star, ring, or bus configured. Local area networks are popular communications networks because they allow for the sharing of computer equipment, resulting in substantial savings in costs

TRENDS IN AUTOMATED OFFICE SYSTEMS

Many of the changes that are in progress in daily business functions are due to communications technology. The applications of both computer and communications technology will continue well into the next decade. Although it may be some time before we actually conduct business in a completely paperless office system, the use of office automation products and services are established practice. Let's explore some of the technology currently in use in offices.

Electronic Mail (E-Mail)

Through the use of a telephone and a modem—along with the appropriate hardware and software—messages, queries, documents, and even graphics are being transmitted electronically. Mail can be stored in a recipient's "mailbox" (a specified location on disk) for receipt at a later time. The receiver can process the mail by reading it, acknowledging and saving, or simply deleting the communication. The main advantages of electronic mail systems within organizations consist of increased productivity for workers. Messages sent can be received by an individual not immediately available to the sender and appropriate responses made at a more convenient time without repeated contact or loss of time through interrupted work.

Voice Mail

Some electronic mail message systems can actually process voice input. These systems are called **voice mail systems**. Voice mail consists of messages sent and stored electronically over a telephone device. Sound waves can be converted into digital code and then stored for retrieval. When the code is retrieved it is then translated back into an audio message. Individuals may retrieve their messages and respond to them at their convenience or during times when peak work hours have passed. Voice mail can be sent to one receiver or a number of recipients at the same time.

Electronic Bulletin Board Systems (BBS). Computers can be used to link up with bulletin board services. Many users of local BBS use these systems to get answers from other users on questions concerning software use.

Facsimile

Facsimile or FAX machines electronically transmit documents over telephone lines to all over the world. The document to be transferred is placed in a FAX machine by the sender, the 'send' button is pressed, and the FAX number of the person receiving the document is dialed. The FAX machine then translates the document into a digital code and sends the code to the FAX machine that is receiving it. The recipient's machine will reproduce the document at the new location.

Teleconferencing

Teleconferencing can be defined as two-way communication between individuals from two or more locations. Teleconferencing systems may transmit voice or voice and visuals (text, graphics, etc.) and can occur between distant locations. It is possible to lease teleconferencing facilities although large corporations may find it cost effective to maintain their own.

Ergonomics

Ergonomics refers to the scientific study of work and space, including the factors that affect worker productivity and that impact on workers' health. Computer manufacturers and furniture companies are developing new and improved working structures to adjust to the automated office and to develop a productive and safe workplace. Techniques for reducing eyestrain have already been discussed in the chapter on input and output devices. Other ergonomic concerns have developed due to office automation. These revolve around questions of the relationship between radiation and disease, and the increase of employee isolation through working predominantly with a computer terminal. These issues are of vital concern to employers and employees alike. It is the responsibility of the companies employing automated technology to address these issues and make adjustments for them.

Telecommuting

Use of communications and computer technology has already had a profound effect on the manner in which business is conducted in the U.S. One unique development, expected to increase rapidly within the next decade, is that of telecommuting (allowing workers the freedom to choose to make their home their base for professional operations). Engineers and telemarketers, accounting personnel and medical transcriptionists—a wide range of professional groups with their own set of responsibilities—are making the changes necessary to assume the challenge of telecommuting.

Since this type of arrangement is relatively new for most modern workers, telecommuting is being seriously studied by management teams and industrial scientists. Policy guidelines for the telecommuter are being written and established and will probably experience many procedural changes over the next few years. Procedures for telecommuters will, of course, vary among the various organizations that offer this option to its employees.

Questions that remain to be studied revolve around issues such as sustaining worker productivity, providing for supervision, maintaining the employee status of the telecommuter, and requirements for employee participation in telecommuting programs.

INFORMATION SERVICES

Information services offers public domain software (freeware), to its users. Information services allow subscribers access through data communications to large data banks. Subscribers to information services pay a fee in order to maintain their access to the data banks. Most information services provide subscribers with access on a 24-hour basis. Rates for access vary across peakload, weekday, and evening time periods. Two of the major information services available for subscription services are The Source and CompuServe. Special interest information services are available for a wide range of professional groups, including health care professionals, Figure 7–1.

CHAPTER SUMMARY

Communications and computer technology have joined forces to allow for the transfer of data and information from one location to another. The term data communications refers to this process. Transmissions can vary according to the type of transmission, the speed of transmission, and the type of channel used to transmit. Factors such as reliability, speed, and cost will influence the decision to choose one mode of transmission over another.

Many changes may occur in the accepted standards for doing business as a result of the technology of data communications. Automated office environments are generating new ways of working including telecommuting, teleconferencing, and the use of electronic and voice mail.

TERMINOLOGY AND REVIEW EXERCISES

Essential Vocabulary

data communications
data transmission
serial transmission
parallel transmission
asynchronous transmission
synchronous transmission
simplex transmission
half-duplex transmission

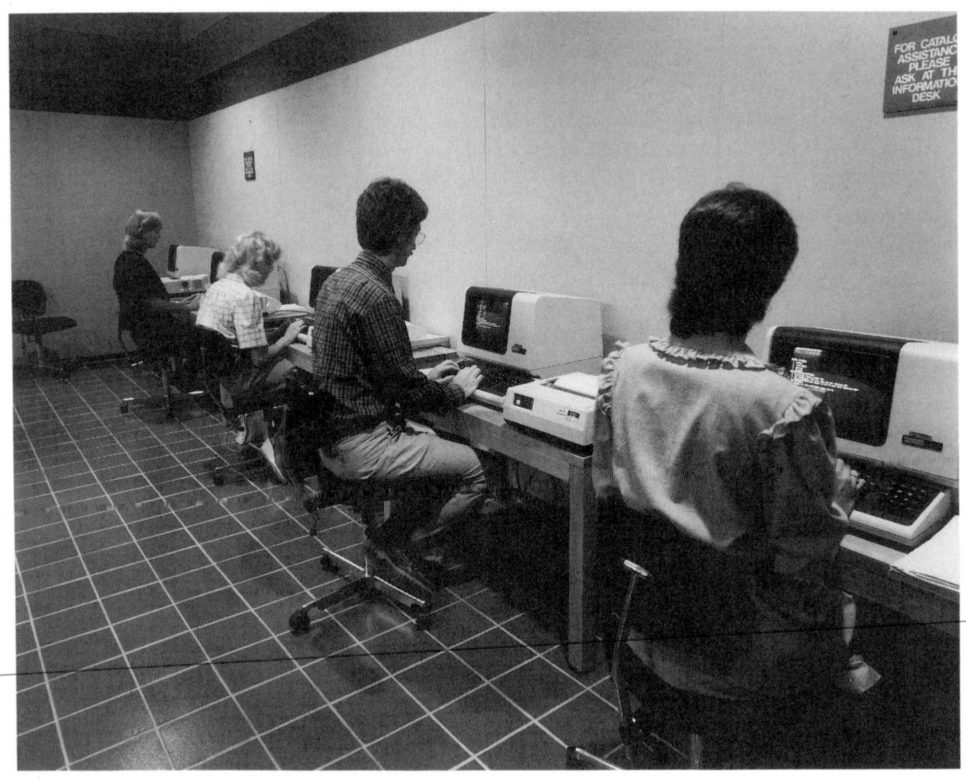

Figure 7–1 The library information system at San Antonio's Dolph Briscoe Library replaces the traditional card catalogue. Users can learn what is available, and whether it is checked out. The system also can connect users to the National Library of Medicine and other data bases to learn of other resources that may be in print. ***(Courtesy of University of Texas Health Science Center, San Antonio, Texas)***

Essential Vocabulary *(continued)*

- full duplex transmission
- bps
- Mbps
- baud
- bandwidth
- narrowband transmission
- voiceband transmission
- broadband transmission
- coaxial lines
- microwaves
- satellite transmission
- communication service carriers
- value added networks
- Telenet
- Tymnet
- modem
- external direct-connect modem
- internal direct-connect modem
- multiplexors
- front end processor
- data communications software
- star configuration
- ring configuration
- bus configuration
- local area networks
- electronic mail systems

voice mail
electronic bulletin boards
facsimile machines
teleconferencing
ergonomics
telecommuting
information services

True/False

1. Serial transmission occurs when data is transferred in groups of bits.
2. Half duplex transmission allows for data to move in both directions simultaneously.
3. Modems are a type of hardware used in data communications.
4. External modems cannot be transferred from one computer system to another.
5. Three types of distributed processing configurations are star, ring, and hierarchical.
6. Local area networks are microcomputers linked by communication lines.
7. Teleconferencing transmits both voice and textual data to distant locations.
8. Electronic mail systems can result in increased productivity for workers.

Fill in the Blanks

1. ______________ ______________ refers to bytes being moved one at a time while ______________ ______________ refers to a group of bytes being moved at one time.
2. Asynchronous transmission moves data by marking a byte of data with a ______________ ______________ and a ______________ ______________.
3. ______________ ______________ is a type of data transmission where data is transferred in one direction only.
4. The most expensive type of transmission line used is a ______________ ______________. It transmits at a line speed of over 9600 bps.
5. Telephone lines, coaxial cables, and satellites are types of ______________ ______________.
6. ______________ refers to the scientific analysis of relationships between work and space.
7. ______________ ______________ transfers voice messages electronically over a telephone device.
8. A FAX machine refers to a device known as a ______________ ______________ which sends duplicates of documents over communication lines.
9. In ______________ ______________ data is transferred by moving all bits in a byte one at a time.
10. Data communications ______________ regulates the transfer of data over communication lines.

Review Questions

1. Distinguish between the three types of data transmission.
2. Differentiate between the types of data communication lines.
3. List and describe the characteristics of the three types of network configurations.

Chapter 8

Administrative Applications in Health Care

Chapter Outline

OBJECTIVES

1. Define administrative, clinical, and special purpose information systems.
2. Identify categories of information required for processing billing for health care services.
3. Identify basic classification systems that facilitate insurance claims processing.
4. Identify basic accounting procedures that are processed through computerized systems.
5. Discuss the role of computerization in cost containment.
6. Define prospective payment and the role it performs in health care financing.
7. Identify operations management procedures that have effectively undergone automation.
8. Discuss the differences between interfaced and integrated computer systems.
9. Identify two experimental computer systems that provide integrated clinical and administrative functions for hospitals and ambulatory care facilities.

TYPES OF COMPUTER APPLICATIONS IN HEALTH CARE

Automated or computerized systems may be employed in administrative, clinical, or special purpose applications.

Administrative Systems

Administrative applications systems in a health care facility include general accounting functions, financial management functions, facilities management, materials management, and general office computer systems.

Clinical Systems

Clinical applications systems can cover a wide range of professional activities and departments as well. Clinical applications are those applications that support patient care. They include automated medical records, nursing care, clinical decision support systems, order entry, and transmission for requested services. Clinical applications enhance patient care by providing information on services that have been provided and by identifying necessary services that may be needed.

Special Purpose Systems

Special purpose systems are systems that provide services other than strictly medical, nursing, and/or administrative. Special purpose systems include laboratory, x-ray, and pharmacy services. Other services that might be considered special purpose in inpatient care facilities might include food service or housekeeping and environmental maintenance.

In this chapter the focus is on administrative functions that have been successfully automated. These functions include general administrative functions and those functions that can be classified under the heading of operations management. Later chapters will examine clinical and special purpose computer systems.

ACCOUNTING AND FINANCIAL MANAGEMENT APPLICATIONS

Billing Systems

Most businesses deliver goods and services to a customer, present their bill, collect their payment, and go on to the next customer. These relatively straightforward procedures just do not apply to the business of providing health care. The complexity of payment for health care services makes computerized billing systems an effective way of managing this particularly cumbersome data processing task.

The variables involved in billing for health services are numerous. Basic questions must be answered before billing for a hospitalized patient can begin to be processed. Billing procedures for ambulatory patients may involve special handling as well. General categories of information include identification of the patient, identification of the insurance carrier or carriers of the patient, and the type of insurance that covers the patient as well as information concerning the physicians that provide care to the patient. Under each of these categories many questions must be answered fully so reimbursement for basic services provided for the patient is guaranteed.

Patient Identification Variables. Patient identification variables include the name of the patient, the patient's social security number, the patient's address and phone number, the patient's employer, and the name of any insurance carriers under which the patient is covered.

Insurance Variables. Patient insurance variables include the identification numbers of insurance policies, the categories of insurance that provide coverage for the patient, and the structure of any private policy that covers the patient. Questions that might require answers include:

- Is the patient insured by a private insurance carrier?
- What does the patient's policy cover?
- Does the patient's insurance require any copayments or deductibles?
- Is there more than one insurance policy?
- What will be covered by which insurance policy?
- Does the patient receive payment directly or can the patient assign (turn over) his benefits directly to the provider?
- Is the patient eligible for coverage under special governmental payment plans such as Medicare, Medicaid, and CHAMPUS?
- Is the patient covered through Workmen's Compensation?
- If there are remaining balances on the bill after all insurance payments have been made, how will the patient pay the remaining portions of the bill?
- If the patient cannot pay a remaining balance, what procedures will be followed?

Provider Variables. Provider variables must also accompany the request for payment of services. These variables may include the name of the physician, an identification number for the provider, and information that the provider must report concerning the classification of the patient, including diagnosis and type of service received.

Office Practice Billing Systems

Health care providers working with ambulatory patients must bill for services. Sometimes these payments involve insurance claims, Medicare or Medicaid claims, or Worker's Compensation. Payments by ambulatory patients can also be made by check or cash. Payments may be made incrementally, with a portion of the total bill being paid monthly. Each of these types of payments for services rendered must be handled appropriately through the billing system mechanism. Computerized systems allow for an efficient means of collecting and processing the data that flows through a typical medical facility, Figure 8–1.

Computerized systems also allow the data processed through billing to become the input for basic accounting functions. Systems that automate billing and accounting functions for a provider are generally referred to as **practice management systems**. These systems can be generalized systems appropriate for various types of practices or they may be practice specific systems that apply only to specialty practices. Practice specific systems can be dental offices, radiology offices, psychiatric practices, or any number of practices that reflect particular processing needs not covered by the general practice systems.

Depending on the size and complexity of the practice, software may be organized into **modules** that provide automated functions at different levels. Modules may consist of subsets

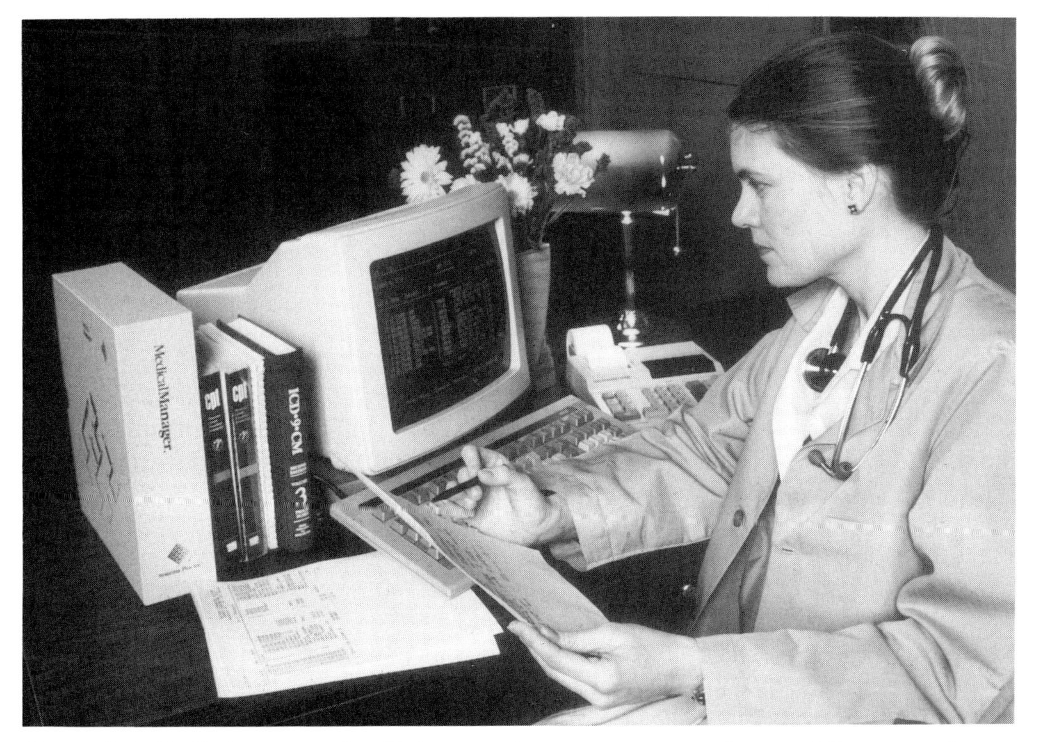

Figure 8–1 Medical personnel utilizing practice management software. ***(Courtesy of Systems Plus, Inc.)***

of software that perform functions such as billing, accounts receivable, and payroll. A modular system provides the advantage of allowing the medical practice to automate in stages. This transitional type of system is useful for growing practices that wish to move to automated systems slowly with little interruption in their daily practice.

Insurance Claims Forms

Most insurance claims forms have been standardized so that the information included in the form can be used to process forms through a number of health care insurance carriers. These claims forms are referred to as **universal claims forms**. The insurance carriers that accept these forms can be either private carriers or government funded programs such as Medicare.

The data required on universal insurance claims forms include the date of service, basic patient information, provider data, information regarding the insurer, the patient's diagnoses, and procedures or tests that have been performed. All the required information must be present on the claim form in order for the provider of the care to receive proper and timely reimbursement. Delays in the processing of claims are largely due to errors on the claim form. Items that have been inadvertently left out may cause the claim to be rejected. Claims that are rejected must be analyzed for the errors they contain and then resubmitted after corrections have been made. These errors can prove costly in terms of the time it takes for employees to reprocess claims and of the lost or delayed reimbursement for procedures already performed. Accuracy and completeness are characteristics that become essential in the processing of claims. Computerized billing systems allow for prompt and reliable submission of insurance claims.

Coding and Computerized Classification Systems. Because of the complexity of health care billing, coding systems have been devised that assist in the processing of claims forms.

DRGs are **Diagnostic Related Groups**. DRGs are codes used in hospitals where the hospital reimbursement is in part determined by the diagnosis the patient receives. DRGs are a cost containment measure and can be used as a quality assessment tool.

ICD-9-CM classifies diseases. This classification system utilizes over 1000 disease categories. **ICD-9-CM** stands for the International Classification of Diseases. This system is recognized as a standard for diagnosis coding and generally consists of a four or five digit code.

CPTs or Current Procedures Terminology codes services such as laboratory tests, examinations, treatments, and operative procedures. These codes allow the provider to enter in the appropriate number along with the description of the procedures performed for that particular patient. The use of these codes facilitates claims processing.

Electronic Claims Processing. Because the processing of insurance claims forms is so vital to the daily financial functioning of the health care facility, **electronic claims processing** has become a common practice among health care providers. Electronic claims processing allows the provider to use a computer with a modem to process "paperless claim forms." These paperless claim forms are sometimes processed through **electronic claims clearinghouses.** The clearinghouse transmits the claim to the appropriate insurance carrier electronically where feasible. If necessary the clearinghouse also prepares a paper claim form and forwards it to the appropriate organization. These electronic claim forms aid health care providers by establishing mechanisms to insure that claims are error free, reducing the number of rejected claims and decreasing the time involved in claim processing. Electronic claims processing allows for **audit trails** to be performed on insurance claims. These audit trails mark and track claims that have not been paid. This particular feature is valuable, saving countless hours searching through files for misplaced or mishandled claims forms.

Computerized Accounting Systems Versus Financial Management Systems

Accounting systems that have been computerized may be part of an overall information system or may be focused on the accounting function alone. Computerized accounting systems may be utilized in hospitals, large teaching facilities, nursing homes, health maintenance organizations, large group practices, or community health programs. These systems generally collect data from a variety of sources that provide input into the system. For example, in a hospital setting the admissions department will provide information on new patients, including basic patient data such as insurance coverage and name of admitting physician.

Accounting systems generally cover applications pertinent to accounts receivable, accounts payable, insurance billing and claims submission, and payroll. **Financial accounting systems** may provide more complex computerized analysis for the provider. They may provide management with statistical data utilized in decision making functions. Some of these systems may support the generation of reports used for budget preparations and forecasting. Reports can also be generated that are linked to the analysis of income by provider or even by piece of laboratory equipment.

Prospective Payment and Cost Containment

Medicare, Part A, provides coverage for hospital services on a **prospective payment** system. This change in health care reimbursement has led to increased interest in developing automated systems that are capable of facilitating the delivery of health care services in a **cost efficient** manner. The trend toward the delivery of health care services through government financing will continue to increase the demand for **cost containment** mechanisms. Because health care costs have increased over the years at an alarming rate, computerized systems that can aid providers in determining the cost effectiveness of health care services are essential.

The prospective payment system allows for the payment of services provided to be determined in advance. The DRGs coding system is linked to the prospective payment system for inpatient hospital services for Medicare recipients. Hospitals are paid in advance based upon the DRG classifications of its patients. When hospitals deliver care within the specified DRG reimbursement formula the hospital is not at risk for financial loss. However, when the care provided to a patient exceeds the amount established, the hospital may be expected to absorb the loss. The DRG based payment formulas may be applied by other providers as well. Because the financial incentive is to reduce unnecessary services, the prospective payment systems may be linked to the provision of quality patient care.

Computerized accounting and administrative applications are the most highly developed systems operating within health care settings. They provide for the basic data processing functions normally found within a business environment.

TRENDS IN HEALTH CARE FINANCING SYSTEMS

Computerized account and financial management systems have been in place and operative for many years. Just within the past decade has the emergence of new technology provided a mechanism for producing up-to-date reliable information at incredible speeds. These changes are responsible for influencing many of the changes taking place within the health care system. The trends in health care provision of the 1990s are toward developing an integration of administrative and clinical systems. While in the past these functions may have seemed directly in conflict, technology is developing the capacity for interlocking and relating the diverse aspects of the health care industry. Ultimately, these integrated computer systems will facilitate information flow both to providers and administrators, enhancing communication at all levels within an organization. The purpose of implementation of new technology within this framework is to ensure quality patient care that is COST EFFECTIVE.

Cost constraints will continue to play a strategic role in the shaping of the health care system within the United States in the years to come.

Physicians, nurses, and other health care professionals may come under scrutiny for the performance of costly procedures that do not significantly alter patient outcomes or improve a patient's health status. Data may be collected and distributed to increase awareness by health care personnel regarding the cost of procedures and practices. Initial research reports this information flow may actually impact positively by reducing unnecessary expense and costly resource consumption.

Even though initially there may be some resistance to health provision changes, the institution of cost effective measures that are also health effective measures does not necessarily have to be a visionary's dream. It can translate into more available dollars that can result in significant improvements in the delivery of health care services to those who are in need.

ASPECTS OF OPERATIONS MANAGEMENT

The day-to-day functioning of a health care facility is a complex combination of operations that must function cohesively to provide a product—the provision of health care services. **Operations management** refers to a branch of investigation that looks at organizations and the way their different departments or groups of personnel perform activities. These professional activities work toward the achievement of the organization's goals for production of services. The purpose of operations management is to devise organizational methodologies to provide efficient means of accomplishing organizational goals. These types of investigations are particularly adaptable to the application of computer technology.

Materials Management

Hospitals, nursing homes, clinics, health maintenance organizations, group practices, and even single-provider practices work daily with the problem of maintaining inventory of frequently used equipment and supplies. With large organizations it becomes cost effective to streamline and computerize operations. Hospitals have departments that act as central supply units, housing and transporting supplies to the various locations within the facility as they are needed. Hospital units usually maintain a supply closet that is periodically examined and restocked. Equipment must be maintained; necessary parts for maintenance are generally housed in the central supply or materials management department. The department may also be in charge of maintaining inventory control data on various equipment located throughout the hospital. Automated systems have functioned effectively to aid in the completion of these activities.

Automated systems that process these types of data consist of various hardware and software. Software for this particular type of operations management activity is generally referred to as **materials management software** or **inventory control software**. Bar code readers are frequently employed as an integral part of the materials management system. The readers may be located in various parts of the hospital or health care facility. They can act to monitor inventory levels in stock rooms so that inventory restocking orders are processed quickly and efficiently. Bar code readers can also be set up to process charges to patients for the supplies that are used. Equipment location, its serial number, and other identifying characteristics can be tracked through automated materials management systems. Requisitions can be automated and then linked with the purchasing functions of the materials management division, allowing reorder forms to be issued when supplies reach preprogrammed levels. Reorder data can also become input data for the accounts payable department.

Staffing and Patient Scheduling

Tremendous advances have been made in technology. We can look forward to interesting and fascinating developments in the applications of computers in the health care industry. Imaginations are at work to develop computer systems that absorb much of the tedious, routine activities that must occur as health care services are delivered.

Talking computer systems that act as scheduling managers are already at work. A system has been developed and is available for commercial application. It works with a microcomputer, voice and data software, and a telephone interface that actually calls the appropriate personnel at various facilities and inquires about available bed space. Beds are tracked through the system and classified according to the type of facility required for the patient, whether the bed is assigned to male or female patients, and other specific categories. When a bed is required for a particular patient, telephone contact may be made with the computer system: the computer system will give the name of the facility with available bed space, its phone number, and the name of the person to contact to arrange admission.

Other systems also function effectively in regulating **patient scheduling**. These systems may be designed to handle either inpatient or outpatient facilities. Hospital information systems may provide mechanisms for preregistration of patients. Information provided by the computer system can facilitate appropriate assignment of personnel according to the patient's needs. Assignment of equipment and scheduling for specialty services (such as operating rooms), may also be also be linked to the hospital information system. Discharge information inputed into the system allows for timely information about availability of facilities for incoming patients.

Ambulatory systems may provide for a computerized "appointment book." Patient scheduling can be classified by provider and by department within a facility, providing useful management information while facilitating the scheduling of patients.

INTERFACING AND INTEGRATING COMPUTER SYSTEMS

While administrative, clinical, and special purpose systems exist, many of these systems are of the stand alone variety. Information is generated within one system and is maintained and utilized within the department where it was generated or transferred to another location where it will be used as input into another system. While no argument exists that these systems have facilitated the achievement of increased productivity and the generation of more reliable data, many administrators and providers alike think that the information availability is not being utilized in an efficient manner. Part of this problem is the fact that technology has accelerated at such an incredible pace that computer systems within a health care facility are added in a piecemeal fashion. Few standards have been generated that allow for different computer systems to communicate and trade data from one system to another. Considerable costs involved in the transfer of data from one system to another have raised the interest of administrators in developing efficient means of communicating data from different computer systems.

The movement toward interfacing and **integration** of computer systems approaches this problem and offers more effective utilization of current technology. **Interfaced systems** allow for the transfer of data from one system to another system. The output from one system may be used as input for the other. Interfacing of data may occur at a specific point in time, on a recurring basis. Hospital charges from the nursing units may be transferred to the hospital patient accounting system at the end of each twenty-four hour period, for example. This type of interfacing would occur in a **batch mode**, with all of the data being transferred from one system to another at that particular point in time. Obviously, interfaced computer systems allow for communication to occur between systems and this communication provides a major advantage. The major drawback among interfaced systems is that the information in one system is not always as current as the information in the other.

Real-time mode data transfer can occur from one computer system to another. This type of interface allows for a faster, more current transfer of data to occur. For example, a clinical order for a laboratory procedure has been prepared on a nursing unit. This order is inputed into the patient care computer system. Once the order has been inputed, an automatic transfer of the patient data to the laboratory system will occur. The obvious advantage of this type of interface is that it is more current than the batch mode data transfer.

Integrated systems utilize a common data base. Because of this common data base, the storage of information is not repeated in different locations from one department to another within a health care facility. The integrated system allows for all information to be current and it allows the data to be accessible. At the present time integrated systems are available that allow for the use of a common data base in a limited number of departments. Fully functional integrated systems are still being researched and developed. Vendors may use the word "integrated" when making sales presentations but few systems actually deliver the concept of true integration.

The HELP System

One experimental integrated computer system is operating at the Latter Day Saints Hospital in Salt Lake City, Utah. This computer system is called the **HELP system**.

In conjunction with the University of Utah, the Latter Day Saints Hospital has been working to develop a comprehensive, integrated computer system that serves both administrative and medical components, including research functions of the hospital.

The implementation of the HELP system has been supported by the National Institute of Health and the National Center for Health Services Research. Over a period of twenty years, the HELP system has moved toward increasing the integration of individual systems. This movement toward integration has produced an effective system that assists both clinical and administrative departments in the provision of health care services.

The administrative functions utilize what is called an admit-discharge-transfer system that employs workstations with computer terminals at various locations throughout the hospital including the emergency room, admitting room, and other departmental locations. Patient scheduling is linked to available beds and the computer system is capable of generating necessary room charges as well as equipment and supply charges for patients. Patient tests are integrated into the systems and billing occurs for testing when test results are recorded. Accounting can generate a current account statement for a patient when needed automatically through the HELP system.

Physician and nurse providers who have used the HELP system have responded favorably to the concept of computerized decision support systems that aid clinical decision making and produce accurate, current, and reliable patient information.

COSTAR System

The **COSTAR system** is another computerized and integrated information system that is undergoing experimental development. COSTAR's focus is on development of information technology for ambulatory care systems. The name, COSTAR, stands for the Computer Stored Ambulatory Record and is being designed to replace current handwritten or document-oriented medical records. The COSTAR system maintains patient data while providing necessary administrative functions for ambulatory-based practices. These medical practices can be simply fee-for-service oriented or prepaid-service oriented as found with health maintenance organizations (HMOs).

Part of this experimental approach revolves around the coding of medical information needed for ambulatory practices. Common complaints and vague presenting problems may not be accommodated by currently used coding systems. COSTAR also attempts to standardize and organize complex medical information through use of a directory. This directory is basically a dictionary of acceptable medical terminology recognized by the COSTAR computer system.

The COSTAR system is supported by a large data base that allows for the access and retrieval of information by different administrative and medical personnel. The COSTAR system has the capability for appointment scheduling, accounts receivable, tracking insurance claims, and other practice management activities while maintaining patient data information. Providers use encounter forms for patient examinations and clerical staff enter the completed forms into the COSTAR computer system.

CHAPTER SUMMARY

Computer applications in health care can be categorized by the functions they perform within the health care setting: administrative, clinical, and special purpose. Administrative applications are concerned with the business operations of the organization. Clinical applications are involved with patient care in a more direct manner. Special purpose applications are specialized systems designed to fulfill a particular function.

This chapter describes the administrative applications that use computer systems. One of the most frequently used applications of computer systems in the health care industry is that of accounting and billing. Automated systems that process accounting and billing data can be found both in large teaching hospitals and small solo practitioners' practices.

With the trend toward cost containment in health care, computer applications can aid in controlling administrative costs so that available funds can be used more directly in patient care. Other administrative applications that use computer systems include materials management, staffing, and patient scheduling.

TERMINOLOGY AND REVIEW EXERCISES

Essential Vocabulary

administrative applications systems
clinical applications systems
special purpose systems
patient identification variables
insurance variables
provider variables
practice management systems
modular software systems
universal claim forms
Diagnostic Related Groups (DRGs)
ICD-9-CM
Current Procedures Terminology
electronic claims processing
electronic claims clearinghouses
audit trail
financial accounting systems
prospective payment
cost effective
cost containment
operations management
materials management software
inventory control software
patient scheduling systems
interfacing computer systems
integrated computer systems
batch mode vs. real-time mode
HELP system
COSTAR system

True/False

1. Clinical applications systems are those automated applications that are directly supportive of patient care.
2. Paperless processing of insurance claims is not electronically feasible at this time.
3. Diagnostic Related Groups code patient diagnoses and are used in an effort to contain escalating costs in health care.
4. Current procedures terminology codes services as well as patient diagnoses for electronic claims processing.
5. Audit trails are implemented to identify insurance claims that have not been paid.
6. Operations management as applied to health care facilities concerns itself with the study of effective and efficient ways to provide health care services to patients.
7. Real-time mode data transfer occurs from one computer system to another by providing communication links between the systems so that current data transfers may be maintained.

8. Truly integrated computer systems that join both administrative and clinical functions within a health care facility are still in experimental stages of development.
9. The COSTAR system is an experimental computer system that provides integration of computer systems for hospitals.
10. The HELP system is an example of the integration that can be achieved between both clinical and administrative functions in health care.

Fill in the Blanks

1. ________ ________ ________ refer to computer systems that automate accounting, financial, and facilities management functions for a health care facility.
2. ________ ________ ________ refer to computer systems that automate laboratory or pharmacy services or other services not considered with strictly clinical or administrative functions.
3. Variables that must be considered when processing insurance claims include ________ ________, ________ ________, and ________ ________ ________ variables.
4. Coding systems currently in use in health care facilities include ________, ________, and ________. The ________ are used in determining prospective payment schedules for hospitals.
5. ________ ________ ________ may be used to automate general practices while ________ ________ ________ may apply only to specialty provider practices such as radiology or psychiatry.
6. ________ ________ ________ allows for insurance claims to be processed electronically. These claims may be processed through a ________.
7. ________ ________ investigates organizations and devises organizational methods to increase productivity and achievement of organizational goals.
8. ________ ________ is concerned with maintaining equipment and supplies for a health care facility.
9. An ________ computer system is one that relies on a single data base to provide data for various data processing activities throughout a health care facility.
10. ________ ________ processing occurs at predetermined times with all data being transferred and processed in that one interval.

Review Questions

1. Define and describe the differences between administrative, clinical, and special purpose computer systems.

2. Discuss the role of automation in facilitating cost containment.
3. Describe operations management and the role it assumes in health care delivery settings.
4. Describe computerized administrative applications for ambulatory practice providers.
5. Discuss the difference between integrated and interfaced computer systems within a health care facility.

Chapter 9

Specialized Information Management Systems in Health Care

Chapter Outline

OBJECTIVES

1. Identify uses of computerized software in the functioning of the inpatient and outpatient pharmacy management.
2. Discuss the concept of the record life cycle.
3. Identify and discuss record management systems terminology as applied to the medical record.
4. Discuss automated technology available for medical laboratories management.
5. Discuss computer based educational systems as applied to patient care.
6. Discuss staff and professional development using computer based instructional systems.
7. Discuss the role of computerization in health care research.

COMPUTERIZED PHARMACY SYSTEMS

Inpatient Pharmacy Systems. Computer software systems can monitor drug treatment dosages, drug-food, or drug-drug interactions, and regulate administration of intravenous preparations.

Dosage systems in hospitals interface between the medical unit where treatment is prescribed and the pharmacy department where treatment dosage is prepared. Ordered medications are prepared and then moved from the pharmacy to the nursing units where they can be administered. The computer system may input medical orders directly from the hospital unit via a terminal linked to the pharmacy department. Another method may require sending a source document from the nursing unit, where the order was prescribed, to the pharmacy where the system input takes place. Output can be represented in the form of medication records kept by the administering personnel and added to the medical record. Output also takes the form of a bill to be added to the patient's account.

Drug Interactions. Computerized hospital information systems can provide information on medications, their individual side effects, and possible interaction effects with food or drugs that the patient may be taking. Private computer subscription services may offer access to data bases that provide more complex **drug interaction** analysis.

Drug interaction programs may be available presently in hospitals and large health care facilities, but few outpatient facilities offer this type of service for their patients at this time. One area that needs development is drug interaction monitoring for geriatric outpatient care. Many older patients see different specialists regularly and are prescribed medications based on specific problems that are monitored by these different specialists. Often there is little or no coordination between physicians and other providers to facilitate effective drug interaction monitoring for these patients. Outpatient drug interaction monitoring is presently being added to some pharmacy services. It is an effective method for screening for potential problems.

Monitoring Intravenous Drug Administration. Computer systems are also available to monitor intravenous **drug administration**. Anesthesiology is one area of medicine where these systems are particularly useful. Computer systems can monitor automatically and reliably over a specified time period, giving feedback when changes occur that need attention by the health care professional.

Outpatient pharmacy systems utilized in retail pharmaceutical supply operations generally consist of a limited data base that can access the patient by name or prescription number. Many of these systems offer itemized drug statements for use by their customers in filing for medical deductions with their yearly income tax return or as documentation for third party reimbursement.

MEDICAL RECORDS MANAGEMENT SYSTEMS

Medical records (the documentation of care provided to the patient), offer a tremendous wealth of data to health care professionals. Medical records serve to document treatment plans, include nursing plans, patient statistics, and the outcomes or progress made in response to treatment provided.

Automation of the medical record has been slow. Several reasons account for this fact. The diversity of material found within the medical record is one of them. Other reasons include the lack of reliable storage media and resistance of health care providers to the computerization of the medical record. However, efforts are proceeding to develop satisfactory means with which to accomplish the storage of the medical data typically found within the medical record into machine readable formats. Various sections of the medical record have already been automated to a certain degree. This trend will accelerate as the technology becomes available with which to store more data effectively at a substantial reduction in cost.

The computerization of the medical record is in progress and offers both tremendous obstacles and tremendous potential. The concept of the computerized medical record is often referred to as the **electronic medical record** or the **automated medical record**. Systems are currently being developed and used in varying capacities. Health care professionals can expect to work with the electronic records in some form or fashion during their careers. It is, therefore, useful to consider aspects of records management as related to the medical record.

The organization of the medical record and the ability of health care professionals to retrieve valuable data from them are of top priority. Information from medical records is used in important research studies. Documentation in the medical records may be used in patient accounting functions. Further, medical records become legal documents that support the patient care received. For these reasons, the proper maintenance and storage of the medical record are essential.

Functionally, we may divide the information within the medical record, the patient data, from the medical record itself. By doing so we can look at aspects of computerized records that differ considerably from one another. Patient data and the documentation of care received fall under the general category of clinical applications while the management of the records themselves can be considered a special purpose application.

Records management systems are systems that provide for the organization and control of records. Records may be defined as any recorded data developed and retained as necessary documentation. Patient data falls within this category. **Patient data** may be viewed as the input in a records management system. The grouping of all information related to a particular patient during a particular period is organized into the patient's medical record. These records may be further categorized as active records and inactive or reference records. **Active records** are records that are referred to frequently or may be currently in use. **Inactive records** are records that, while they are not currently in use, need to be maintained for reference purposes such as research data or for legal support.

All records pass through stages of a **record life cycle**. Data originates from various sources or locations and becomes input into the record itself. The **input stage** is the first stage of the record life cycle. Input data may originate from inside or outside the organization where the record is maintained. Input may include forms, dictated and typewritten material, handwritten notes, and other materials.

Within a hospital setting input into the medical record may originate from both within the hospital and from outside it. That is to say, medical consultation reports or *past* patient histories may be forwarded on a particular patient; these reports become part of the patient's *current* medical record. Reports from laboratory analysis, from pathology departments, and from the nursing unit itself all become input into the medical record.

Medical Records Input. Medical records receive input from a variety of sources:

- Orders from physicians and notes from nurses

- Laboratory results
- a variety of other test results.

The record becomes a complex document that reflects a multitude of decisions and actions taken to provide proper medical care.

Processing is the second stage of the record life cycle and includes distribution and production aspects for the record. **Distribution** functions allow individuals within an organization access to the needed material within the record. Encoders need access to the record in order to process insurance claims form. Encoders are responsible for DRG and ICD-9 coding of a patient's record. Others include providers of care and those who assist in the documentation of that care, including unit clerks, medical transcriptionists, and medical secretaries. **Production** functions revolve around how the record is to be used: decision making, referencing, and documenting. Both encoding and transcription functions can both be considered necessary production functions.

Maintenance is the third stage within the record life cycle and is concerned with the storage and retrieval of the record. **Storage** requires the proper placement of the record with an appropriate filing system. **Retrieval** requires determination of the location and physical access to the record.

Active and inactive records may differ in the type of maintenance they receive. Active records will be located within the medical care environment, making quick retrieval and access possible. Inactive records may have their own location, still providing access, with an increased retrieval time.

Disposal is the fourth and final stage of the record life cycle. Records must periodically be removed from the record system. These records serve no viable purpose for the organization and therefore may be discarded according to some predetermined schedule. This schedule is called the **records retention schedule**. Methods of disposal will vary according to the type of material contained within a particular record. Sensitive data may require special handling. Disposal of medical records must be handled with care.

Several areas of controversy surround the issue of computerized patient data and automated medical records. These include confidentiality, data security, retrievability, viruses, and testing to ensure adequacy of information. Discussion of these issues will occur in a later chapter.

Available computer systems can handle a wide range of data from or about medical records. Software programs are available that provide a means for keeping track of medical records. Often these software programs are referred to as **record tracking systems** or **record logging systems**. The medical record is logged *into* the system and can be tracked *with* it. These tracking programs keep track of where the records are, when they are due back, and what records are overdue. Records can be sorted by patient name or I.D. number and overdue reports printed. Bar codes may be used to mark records and charts may be "checked in or out" of the medical records department while the software program tracks its movement.

Other medical records systems offer more complex features such as tracking deficiencies in patients' charts, or organizing deficiencies by physician or department while keeping track of the location of the record. Deficiencies can be noted by category: records requiring physician signature or records requiring completion or dictation.

Software has been developed that allows for computer preparation of various documents that make up the medical record.

Encoding software is available that allows for the classification of patient diagnoses according to ICD-9-CM standards. Some software packages also group patient data into the appropriate DRG categories. This type of automation promotes timely payments through assisting the coding personnel in establishing proper classification of patient information.

Trends in Medical Record Maintenance

Optimally the computerized medical record will be a means of ascertaining important clinical data as well as determining effective treatment modalities along with cost effectiveness.

Classification systems of the future may not be restricted to cost reimbursement mechanisms. They may be directly related to quality assurance and provision of optimal medical care.

Storage systems for permanent medical records in the future will probably use **optical disk storage**. They can provide access to medical records information to authorized users. Additionally, optical disk systems provide an on-line record to capture data automatically from various input sources within the facility or even from remote locations. The information on the disk will be digital. Since optical disk technology is relatively new, the exact legal status in terms of admissibility in a court of law has not been determined. However, anticipation of its acceptance is strong since it meets the strict requirements of reliability and accuracy that are suggested as guidelines for admissibility. Optical disk technology has the benefits of decreasing the amount of storage space required for long term maintenance of medical records. The cost of implementation of optical disk storage will initially be high but promises long term savings in costs of personnel, storage space, and supplies.

Other new technologies that will facilitate the establishment of an electronic medical record are voice recognition and medical text processing. Voice recognition systems are already in use in some specialized departments within hospital systems.

COMPUTERIZED LABORATORY MANAGEMENT SYSTEMS

Laboratory software systems can be management oriented or clinically oriented. **Laboratory management** software has been designed and implemented for both hospital and commercial laboratories. Hospital versions generally include reporting systems that provide for labeling functions, worklist schedules, patient statistical reports, and billing. The software usually can interface with automated analyzers, generating necessary reports. Laboratory software can be linked to the hospital information system. Linked systems provide additional benefits through the provision of access to admission, discharge, and transfer data. Lab orders can be received directly by the lab and results can be reported directly to nursing stations when requested. Lab software systems generally provide for invoicing functions, statements, and lab test results.

COMPUTERIZED INSTRUCTIONAL SOFTWARE SYSTEMS

Computer-based education (CBE) uses computers as an instructional medium. Computers are a potentially valuable medium for instructional purposes because they offer some unique characteristics:

- Computers can work with learners at their own individual rate.
- There is no limitation on how much time a learner can spend on a particular topic or unit of instruction.
- The learner can stay with the instructional program long enough to actually assimilate and master new material.
- Basically, the computer is a machine that can offer a learner a nonjudgmental environment in which to assimilate new information.
- Computers also can test and provide immediate feedback to the learner to give an accurate assessment of the level of mastery.
- Computers offer flexibility to a learning environment that is not readily available in the more traditional sense.

The advantages of computer-based education are numerous: however one disadvantage is obvious. The cost involved in providing a computer learning environment is substantial and remains somewhat prohibitive.

Computer assisted instruction (CAI) includes those instructional models that are concerned with the delivery of basic skills and the acquisition of knowledge by utilizing current computer technology. Computer assisted instruction software employs various instructional strategies and techniques. These software packages include drill and practice, tutorial, simulation, and basic problem-solving.

Drill and practice computer-assisted instruction packages are software packages that offer repetitive question and answer sessions. This type of program is appropriate for educational instruction when rote memorization is required. It has been employed to instruct in basic mathematical skills, foreign language vocabulary development, and computer terminology. Questions can be organized in a fixed sequential pattern or can be accessed randomly.

Drill and practice CAI offers an effective means of providing learners with the practice necessary for basic skills acquisition. Drill and practice software provides a reliable means for assessing mastery level. Scores may be kept on drill and practice CAI programs. Usually the computer keeps track of the number of correct responses for each section completed by the student.

Simulations are computer assisted instructional programs that provide the student with a learning experience that closely resembles what occurs in a real life setting, Figure 9–1. This type of computer assisted instruction is valuable for training in job-related skills that may be too dangerous for the learner to attempt until basic skills are achieved. Flight training uses computer simulation and some teenagers are now learning to drive an automobile using computerized simulation programs.

Problem-solving computer assisted instruction programs allow the learner to apply problem solving methodologies to a particular situation in order to create appropriate solutions. Variables can be selected and tested for their impact upon the simulated situation.

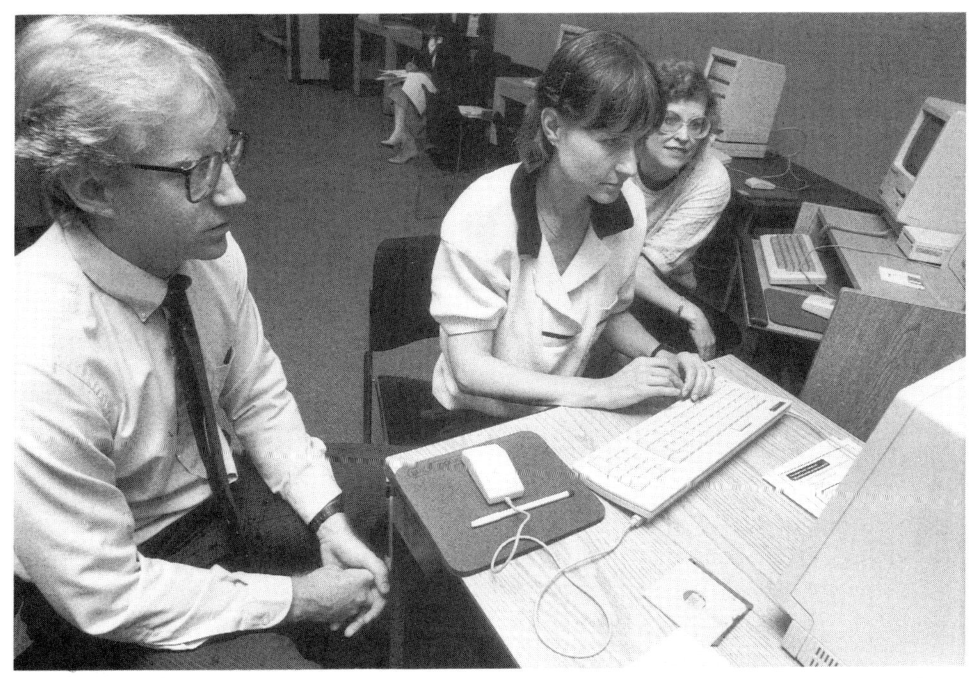

Figure 9–1 Computer terminals located at the University of Texas Health Science Center library allow students to learn by using faculty developed software packages. These software packages allow students to learn by interactive "games" such as an emergency medicine simulation in which students diagnose. ***(Courtesy of University of Texas Health Science Center, San Antonio, Texas).***

Tutorials are a type of computer assisted instruction. Generally, this type of software offers a more advanced application of drill and practice type of instruction. Tutorials often allow the learner to proceed from the basic to the complex at their own rate. Information may be presented in the tutorial; then the user is asked to complete drill and practice sections over the presented material. The tutorial frequently allows the user to return to various levels of instruction to repeat more basic sections of the program. Tutorials differ from drill and practice instructional methodologies in that they seek to test understanding of *concepts* as well as test for simple *memorization.* Movement in a tutorial is from drilling for very basic educational constructs to more complex levels of testing for comprehension.

Computer assisted instructional systems are being developed for both patients and professionals. Patients are receiving instruction that will facilitate their well-being. Professionals are learning through the use of computer technology to function knowledgeably and effectively in providing health care.

Computer-assisted Instruction for Patients. Patients are now becoming involved in a variety of computer assisted instructional systems. Computer systems offer the patient the advantage of not being constricted by time pressures or rigorous schedules of health providers. The computer program can test the patient for basic understanding of the principles being presented. The patient can feel more secure in answering the computer because no human judgment or evaluation is taking place. Further, computer systems can provide the patient with individualized instructions that can be used to follow prescribed treatment regimens. Educational computer programs act to insure proper patient compliance with the recommended procedures.

Patient-oriented computer assisted instruction systems have been developed in the health education area with tutorial software programs instructing patients on fitness regimens such as diet and exercise. These types of programs can be beneficial to patients with high-blood pressure or weight problems. They can assist the patient in behavior modification that can result in significant changes in health status. Other health education programs can center on concerns about teenage alcoholism, raising self-esteem, drug education, tobacco addiction, and AIDS information.

Disease management or patient self care is another area that has successfully established the use of computer assisted instruction for patients. Patient management of diabetes has been developed as a computer assisted instructional tutorial. Pediatric care employs software training instruction for parents in the management of common infections and diseases of their children. Most of these programs offer a hard copy set of instructions that serves to reinforce learning that has occurred during the use of the tutorial program.

Computer Assisted Instruction for Professional Training. Software development for the student and the continuing education of the professional have developed considerably and offer a broad spectrum of modalities. Tutorials and drill and practice programs have been developed for use in medical training programs. These software tools offer the student opportunities to expand their professional training beyond simple classroom and practicum experience.

ILIAD is a commercial computer based educational program designed to teach clinical problem solving skills. It is currently in use in teaching hospitals and universities. This computer program can operate in a simulation mode by offering hypothetical cases for evaluation by the student. While the student evaluates the cases presented, complex medical decision making skills are learned. ILIAD is also capable of determining the level of diagnostic capability of the student by comparing the student's workup with its own response to the hypothetical patient. ILIAD is an example of the commercial applications that have resulted from the investigation of artificial intelligence, which will be presented in later chapters.

HEALTH CARE RESEARCH INFORMATION SYSTEMS

The changes in available technology in computer hardware has had an impact upon how research is conducted within the health sciences field, Figure 9–2.

These changes will continue bringing the potential for rapid advancement in information in a number of disciplines. Increased processing speeds allow for scientific hypotheses to be formulated and tested in a relatively short time span. The generation of large data

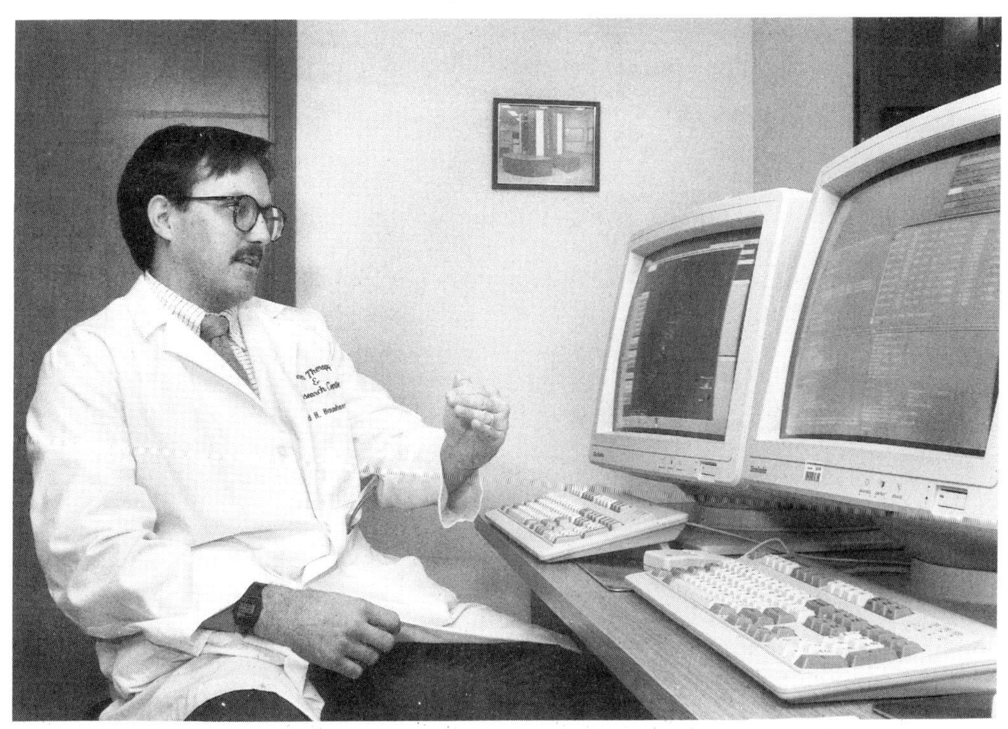

Figure 9–2 Cancer specialist Dr. Frederick H. Hauscheer is using computer technology to design and test new cancer drugs. He uses the computer to recreate a three-dimensional structure of a cell and simulates the manner in which drugs bind or react chemically. ***(Courtesy of University of Texas Health Science Center, San Antonio, Texas)***

banks with incredible storage capacities will also allow for exploration into quite complex inquiries. Some of these trends are occurring now and many will develop in the years to come.

One area where obvious gains have been accomplished is that of information identification and retrieval. Presently it is possible to connect with information retrieval systems and reference topics in the health sciences literature automatically. Most medical libraries and many hospitals have the capacity to use the **MEDLARS** (Medical Literature Analysis and Retrieval Systems) literature data base. This data base, through the National Library of Medicine, allows researchers to conduct literature reviews on any of their twenty on-line bibliographies. One example of their data bases is the BIOETHICSLINE that contains references pertaining to religious, philosophical, and legal issues. Another is **MEDLINE** (Medical Literature Analysis and Retrieval System On Line) that contains over 6 million references on journal articles relevant to health care professionals.

Information systems that complete biomedical journal searches are also becoming available on subscription services to individual purchasers for use on their microcomputers, at their office, or homes. These subscription services periodically mail out floppy diskettes that contain the table of contents from current issues of major journals in biology and medicine. MEDLINE subscriptions are also available for the microcomputer. The individual purchasers access the system across communication lines.

Specialized Prepackaged Software. Software packages are now being produced that allow the user to apply specially designed research programs and to analyze their data using microcomputers. Drug trials are one of the areas where these specialized software packages have been utilized. These **research systems software** packages assist in assuring good research design, data management, and monitoring for pharmacological trials.

Grant management software is available for supporting grant allocation of funds. Expenses are inputed into the system and the software aids in the administration of grant funds.

More general prepackaged systems are also currently available in the marketplace. Statistical packages that allow the user to analyze data on microcomputers is now frequently used within research facilities. Analysis may be made using simple descriptive statistics or more complex formulations. These packages may include color presentation graphics that can assist the researcher in presenting findings in a concise manner.

CHAPTER SUMMARY

Many information management systems are used in health care applications. Most have been designed to automate one particular function within a health care facility.

Computerized pharmacy systems are being utilized in hospitals and research institutions. These computerized systems assist the pharmacy department in tracking medications for patients or analyzing drug-drug or drug-food interactions that may prove harmful to the patient.

Medical records management systems are in the process of being developed. Tracking systems have been introduced that aid in the process of locating records that have been removed from the medical records department.

Laboratory management systems are used to run analyses on blood samples and to track results of testing procedures. The introduction of these systems has proven to be cost effective.

Instructional software is being developed to teach students the fundamentals of care in many of the health care professions. Other types of instructional software relate directly to the patient and use the computer as an patient education tool.

Research institutions are utilizing computer systems to analyze research data. Information is available to researchers using data bases to access new research studies and findings.

TERMINOLOGY AND REVIEW EXERCISES

Essential Vocabulary

dosage systems
drug interaction systems
drug administration systems
electronic or automated medical record
patient data
active records
inactive or reference records
record life cycle
input stage
processing stage

maintenance stage
disposal stage
records retention schedule
record logging and tracking
encoding software
patient data management
optical disk storage
laboratory management systems
computer-based education
computer assisted instruction (CAI)
drill and practice software
simulations software
problem solving software
tutorial software
ILIAD
MEDLARS
research systems software
MEDLINE
grant management software
BIOETHICSLINE

True/False

1. Pharmacy software systems may provide information on drugs and their interactions with other drugs or foods.
2. Automated and electronic are used synonomously when referring to medical records systems.
3. Record management systems are organizational devices that provide for the control of medical records.
4. Reference records are active records that are referred to frequently and are currently in use.
5. The record life cycle originates in the medical records department.
6. Processing is the third stage of the record life cycle and includes distribution and processing functions.
7. A record tracking system is a computer software program that functions with computer hardware to provide data on where records are located and which records are overdue.
8. Encoding software aids in the classification of diseases into appropriate DRG and ICD-9 codes.
9. The exact legal status of optical disk technology in conjunction with its use in storing medical records has been firmly established.

Fill in the Blanks

1. ____________________-__________________ ______________________________ has been successfully developed for staff and professional development as well as for patient self-care.
2. ____________________________ are computer-assisted instructional systems that provide a learning experience similar to what actually happens in a real health care setting.
3. ____________________ is the name of a commercial computer-based educational software program designed to teach clinical problem-solving skills.
4. __________________ and __________________ computer programs provide repetitive question and answer sessions appropriate for learning through memorization.
5. ______________________________ is the third stage of the record life cycle and is concerned with the storage and retrieval of the record.

6. ______________ ______________ ______________ aid hospital and commercial laboratories in the processing of data related to schedules, billing, worklists, and statistical reports.
7. ______________ ______________ ______________ are capable of referencing topics within a bibliographic literature data base. ______________ is a data base that references medical literature and is developed through the National Library of Medicine.
8. The ______________ ______________ ______________ consists of four stages from the records initial ______________ stage to its ______________ stage.
9. Disposal of records is accomplished according to a ______________ ______________ ______________.

Review Questions

1. Describe processing, distribution, and maintenance functions for the medical record. List some of the activities that are related to each function.
2. Discuss the types of software available for use in pharmacies and laboratories.
3. Describe the advantages of using computer-assisted instruction for patient education and disease management.
4. Describe the advantages of using computer-assisted instruction in the training of health care professionals.
5. Discuss some problems associated with automating the medical record.

Chapter 10

Direct Patient Care and Treatment Applications

Chapter Outline

OBJECTIVES
HEALTH ASSESSMENT SYSTEMS
CLINICAL MONITORING AND SPECIAL PURPOSE SYSTEMS
ISSUES IN THE USE OF AUTOMATED SYSTEMS
CHAPTER SUMMARY
TERMINOLOGY AND REVIEW EXERCISES

OBJECTIVES

1. Discuss general and problem specific health assessment systems.
2. Present clinical monitoring systems presently used in critical care environments.
3. Define sensor technology and automated medical instrumentation systems.
4. Discuss pulmonary monitoring systems used in respiratory therapy.
5. Discuss clinical monitoring systems used in obstetrical and neonatal units.
6. Discuss computerized special purpose systems including drug administration systems.
7. Identify and discuss the issues involved in computerized clinical and special purpose systems.
8. Discuss reliability and validity in relation to computerized clinical and special purpose systems.

HEALTH ASSESSMENT SYSTEMS

Health assessment, the determination of a patient's health status, aids the health care provider in determining the patient's need for health care services. Effective assessment can result in identification of patient health problems, identification of risk factors that predispose an individual to develop a particular health problem, or can aid providers in the determination of the most effective treatment or management of health problems. Health assessment computer software facilitates determination of a patient's health status and identification of existing or potential health problems.

Health assessment systems can be categorized into problem specific assessments or general assessments. **General health assessment systems** have been developed to provide a health screening mechanism. With these systems the patient interacts with the computer hardware and inputs answers to simple questions concerning family history, social history, personal habits, and past illnesses.

One advantage of this type of screening is that it allows the patient to answer questions without the attention of a health care professional. This advantage results in cost and time savings because it frees up professional time for other activities.

The second advantage relates to the belief that some patients will react to the computer system by responding in a more complete and reliable manner. Personal questions presented by a health care professional may result in the patient responding in a guarded or reticent manner. Answering questions by machine sometimes results in a more accurate description of the habits impacting on health status.

Both benefits combined add up to a solid foundation for pursuing the study of the actual effectiveness of health assessment software. Preliminary data suggest that computerized screening and health assessment systems can provide a cost effective means of identifying health care problems and patient needs.

Various manufacturers create products that can be classified as general health assessment or health screening software. The software capabilities range from identifying health risks in individuals, assigning a health age, preparing a report that predicts age expectancy based on the patient's health assessment, and suggesting methods of prolonging life expectancy by modifying behavior.

Problem specific health assessment software identifies risk factors for specific types of health problems. Cardiology systems may test for risk of coronary artery disease by analyzing patient data taken during stress exercise testing. Cardiology assessment is perhaps the most sophisticated of the problem specific software and several manufacturers offer this type of software for purchase.

Problem specific health assessment software is generally developed for patient screening within a particular specialty area. Patients may answer questions during initial interviews by responding to symptoms shown individually on the computer system's monitor. Software packages are available for subspecialty areas such as endocrinology, urology, ophthalmology, and pulmonology. Problem-specific software may also assess patient data through a question and answer system designed with an answer format such as yes/no or multiple choice.

Problem specific assessment may occur for a variety of patient problems. Examples of available software include patient nutrition analysis for providing patients with nutritionally balanced meals or to guide patients in a clinically directed weight loss program. Other types of software may provide patient analysis for areas such as obstetrical patient management and occupational health screening.

CLINICAL MONITORING AND SPECIAL PURPOSE SYSTEMS

Computerized clinical monitoring systems are computer systems that regularly provide surveillance and reporting functions for individual patients. Major types of clinical monitoring systems are **physiological**, **arrythmia**, **pulmonary**, and **obstetrical/neonatal**. These computer systems evaluate input from the patient directly, analyze the patient data, and organize the data into meaningful form, Figure 10–1.

Clinical services and computerized applications involve direct provision of health care services to the patient. These clinical applications may include physiological monitoring systems, arrhythmia monitoring systems and other diverse special purpose systems. Many of these systems are operating within critical care environments using sensor technology.

Special purpose systems are computer systems facilitating particular aspects of patient care. The special purpose systems include drug administration systems, patient maintenance systems such as the Holter monitor, and rehabilitative systems designed for disabled individuals.

Sensor Technology

Clinical monitoring may take place with the aid of a **sensor** or **sensing device**. Sensors are compact, high performance devices adapted to the particular data requirements. Sensors detect minute changes in measurements such as temperature, pressure, or other physiological measurements. **Transducers** convert the basic signals picked up by the sensing device into other, more readable forms. These measurements in turn may be used to calculate and produce output through a central processing unit.

Signal processing units include components necessary to produce the required output. These components generally include the sensing device, signal conditions or transducers, display devices, a central processing unit, and a controller. Signal conditioners alter or filter the initial input picked up by the sensing device to make the output easier to read or evaluate. Display devices can be cathode ray tubes or monitors displaying graphics. Printers are also display devices, documenting all available output with a hard copy printout. The central processing unit of the signal processing system is the microprocessor that completes the logical and computational processing tasks.

Automated signal processing units or signal analysis systems perform various functions depending on the complexity of design. Fundamentally,

- They collect and evaluate data to provide information on a patient's health status.
- They may function to provide surveillance and recognition mechanisms for predetermined values. Frequently they may analyze, evaluate, or interpret the input data they receive.
- Input data may be used to provide output for human analysis in either the same form or the data may be modified in some way.
- Automated systems can store the output data for future reference.
- They produce hard copy documentation for entry into the patient's medical record.

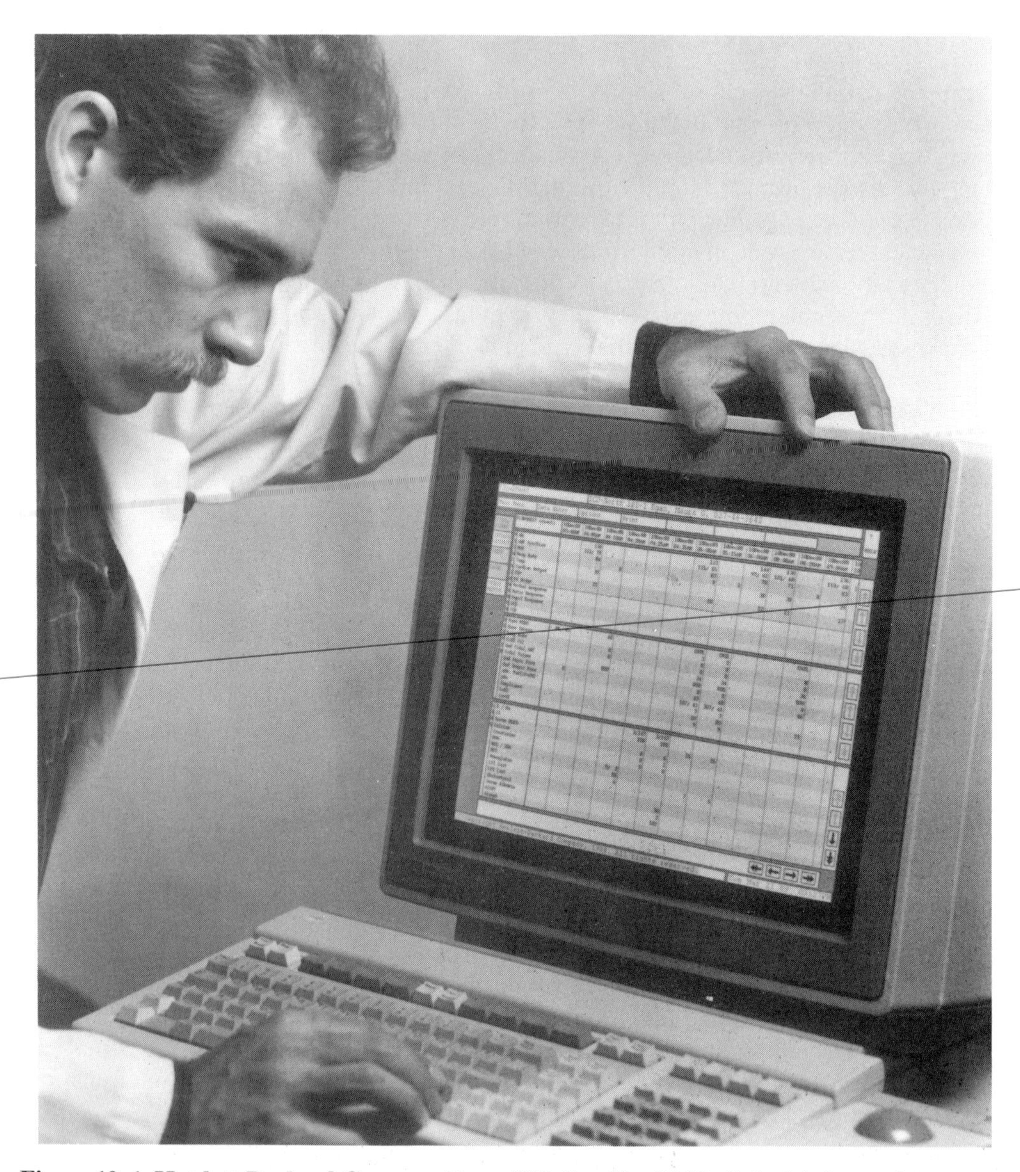

Figure 10–1 Hewlett-Packard Company's new HP CareVue 9000 clinical-information system is a bedside-oriented system designed to replace and automate the charting process in the critical-care area of the hospital. Its powerful bedside work stations collect information from patient monitors and other bedside devices and integrate it with important observation data. ***(Courtesy of Hewlett-Packard Company)***

Feedback Control Mechanisms. When monitoring systems provide control mechanisms that respond appropriately to the monitored condition of a patient, these control mechanisms may be either closed or open loop systems. Engineers, health care providers, and computer programmers cooperate in an interdisciplinary effort to develop computerized medical instrumentation.

Other terms used in reference to signal processing units are computerized or **automated medical instrumentation**. These terms refer to medical instruments or equipment that operate through electronic means to provide input via measurements, perform data collection and data analysis tasks. Drug administration systems that control the amount of drug administered are an example of automated medical instrumentation. Another example of automated systems would be that of the electrocardiogram systems continuously monitoring and recording data on the patients in an intensive care environment.

Critical care environments. Automated operating rooms, emergency rooms, and intensive care environments assist providers of care in determining rapidly and accurately those patients who require attention. It is important for health care professionals to develop an awareness of the potential for computerization in these areas since these environments have become highly technological in design and function.

Since patients in the intensive care units or those undergoing surgical or emergency procedures require special care, technology simplifying the delivery of that care is extremely useful. By becoming aware of how these computer systems operate, future applications will be developed that aid in the delivery of health care.

Physiological Monitoring Systems

Physiological monitoring systems are computer systems that monitor physical processes, such as analyzing blood or other fluids. These systems sometimes alert staff when levels reach a need for clinical action. Monitoring systems track physiological processes, graphing or charting data to provide necessary documentation of the physical process under observation. Sometimes alarm systems may be triggered when certain predetermined changes in patient status occur. These alarm systems aid providers in assessing patient health status.

The advantages of computerized physiological monitoring systems are numerous. Time that was once spent in data collection through repeated measurements and documentation of those measurements is now free for other more direct patient care activities. The data collected through automated systems is more reliable. With properly serviced and functioning equipment, automated systems provide fast and accurate measurements that can be easily documented. Hard copy documentation can be delivered for placement into a medical record or a CRT display can provide a visual report to the observations collected. Automated instrumentation can analyze certain types of information and help to organize data for providers to evaluate. Analysis by computerized systems can result in identification of life-threatening problems. Problem identification frequently aids in appropriate decision making and treatment by the health care team, Figure 10–2.

Physiological monitoring systems can be classified by the data processing components of the system. Input functions involve a basic data gathering system usually accomplished through some type of sensor that collects the required data. Once the data has been collected, processing can occur in many ways. Mathematical operations may occur on the data or the data may be altered in another way (through amplification). Data may be classified or categorized in some manner during the processing. Once processing has occurred, output

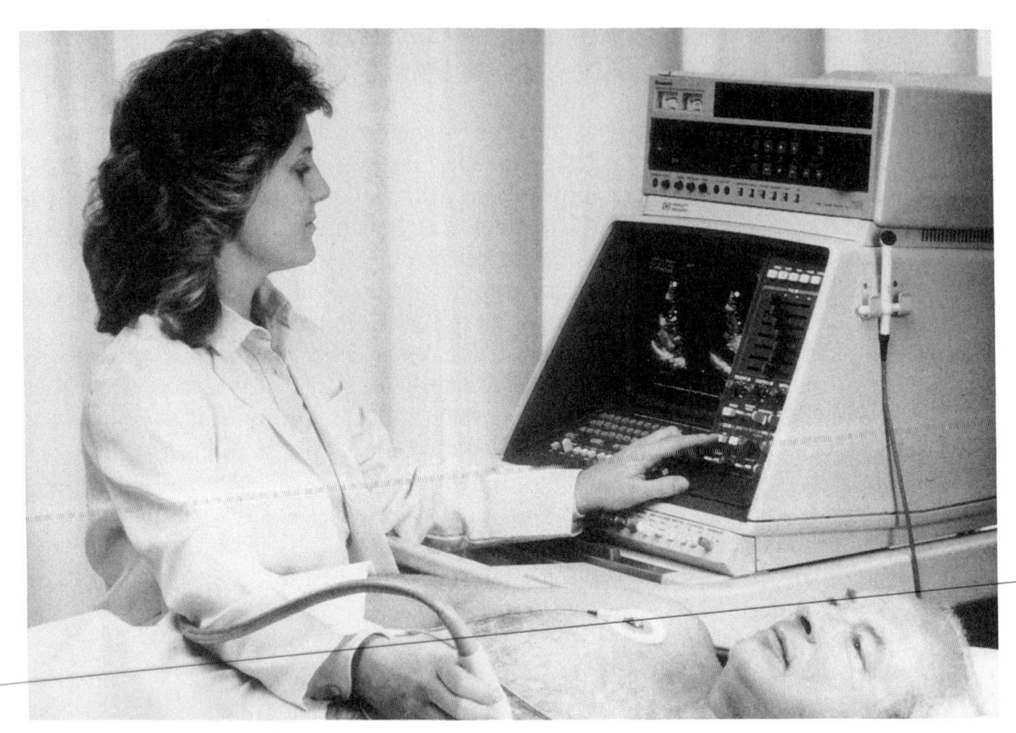

Figure 10–2 The HP SONOS 1000 cardiovascular imaging system from Hewlett-Packard is designed for demanding, high-performance imaging requirements. New precision-imaging electronics and 128-element transducers with frequency agility deliver sensitive Doppler and color flow without compromising high resolution cardiac images. ***(Courtesy of Hewlett-Packard Company)***

can take place. Examples are hard copy reports, visual representations on a screen, or alerts that require further evaluation and action. Self regulating systems may provide mechanisms for actions to be implemented automatically by the monitoring system itself, in effect, carrying out a preprogrammed treatment regimen.

Many physiological monitoring systems are now manufactured and produced in a modular format, with one piece of equipment being added to another to increase the system's potential. These modular physiological monitoring systems are frequently called **patient bedside monitors** or **bedside patient management systems**. These bedside monitors offer noninvasive, continuous monitoring of patients in critical care areas.

Patient bedside systems are integrated computer systems since they allow for more than one function to be performed such as physiological and respiratory monitoring. These systems generally allow for nurses to enter or input clinical observations and relevant laboratory data. Data organization and data management functions are performed by the system.

Some patient bedside management systems allow for linkage and communication to occur with a larger host computer, allowing for a reduction in data replication. In experimental stages it is also possible for physicians to complete rounds and consultations from remote monitor screens without attending the patient at the bedside.

Arrhythmia Monitoring

Another standard type of computerized medical instrumentation is the arrhythmia monitor, used in emergency rooms, operating rooms, and intensive care areas. Arrhythmia monitors provide basic monitoring or diagnostic support for patients. These monitors increase the detection of fatal arrhythmias by monitoring heart rates. The systems detect when heart rates fall out of a preprogrammed range; they have demonstrated the potential of reducing mortality for patients experiencing severe coronary problems.

Arrhythmia systems may even provide diagnostic capabilities that can be evaluated through communications with an off-site cardiologist. When computer systems involve diagnostic capabilities, the diagnosis made may be called a **computer-assisted diagnosis**. The computer system performs a rhythm analysis and then reports a diagnosis resulting from the analysis. The computer is preprogrammed to interpret the data and results in reliable diagnostic information.

Arrhythmia monitoring systems provide similar advantages that apply to physiological monitoring systems. They reduce clerical activities for the nursing personnel and increase the time nursing staff can spend in other patient care activities. In addition to aiding in the diagnostic evaluation of the patient, these systems produce necessary documentation in a clear and concise format.

Arrhythmia monitoring systems are manufactured by several well established and reliable corporations, including IBM and Hewlett-Packard. Usually arrhythmia monitoring systems are **dedicated computer systems**. Dedicated systems are computer systems designed for processing information for a single or special purpose, in this case, patient monitoring. Arrhythmia monitoring systems collect data on the activity of the heart, blood pressure, and heart rate. These systems provide continuous monitoring of a patient's condition and can provide feedback to nursing staff and other providers when the patient's heart rate is outside normal, acceptable limits.

Pulmonary Monitoring Systems

Respiratory therapy requires the precise measurements of pulmonary flow, gas concentrations, and respiratory rates. Automated systems deliver these measurements continuously for patients in intensive care environments or provide short-term monitoring, supporting diagnostic evaluation of respiratory therapy patients.

Respiratory patients may be tested for pulmonary function with automated systems that analyze patients under stress test conditions. **Turnkey respiratory function systems** provide complete pulmonary function analysis. These systems are capable of testing (including spirometry and lung-volume tests), providing automated calibration, and displaying pre- and post-bronchodilator graphic comparisons.

Testing for respiratory functions may involve pneumotachographic recorders that assess respiratory volume and rate. Other respiratory measurements include airway flow, pressure, and gas concentrations. From baseline measurements taken, further calculations may be made that can be used to interpret patient status or condition. Respiratory measurements and calculations can be effectively performed by computerized medical instrumentation.

Obstetrical and Neonatal Monitoring Systems

Physiological monitoring has been implemented and utilized successfully in obstetrical and neonatal care units. Neonatal or newborn nursery units may have monitoring systems that provide continuous surveillance and detection for an infant's heart rate and respiratory rates. Such monitoring systems can provide detection for apnea or respiratory arrest and may aid in the prevention of the mortality associated with such arrest.

Obstetrical personnel may monitor interuterine pressure during oxytocin therapy using automated equipment. Use of the automated monitoring system reduces the oxytocin necessary to produce dilation and the amount of oxytocin can be regulated by the system to reduce or stop oxytocin levels at signs of either fetal distress or hypercontractility. High risk pregnancies are carefully monitored through fetal heart rate monitoring during labor. This type of monitoring is standard treatment for patients experiencing problem pregnancies.

Monitoring of neonates occurs continuously using the cardiorespirography method to detect alarm parameters in either heart rate or respiratory rates. While cardiorespirography provides a method of continuous monitoring, the testing mechanism currently reflects less than 100% validity.

Drug Administration Systems

Anesthetic administration may be accomplished through the use of vaporizers. These **vaporizers** convert liquids into a gaseous form so that inhalational anesthesia may be administered. During administration the amount of gas administered must be closely supervised. Patient monitoring also occurs during the administration of anesthesia and documentation of the process must occur. Experimental studies using **infusion pumps** show their potential for treatment of hypertension, management of intractable pain, and other applications, including cancer therapy.

Patient Maintenance Systems

A somewhat new class of automated medical instrumentation systems allow for the complete maintenance of a patient concerning some aspect of their care. **Patient maintenance systems** are generally a type of special purpose systems that offers complete automation of some aspect of patient care. These systems are still largely experimental and their study and development proceeds under carefully controlled research conditions. These automated patient maintenance systems control the level of anesthesia delivered to a patient; controls substance infusion such as drugs, dye or blood; and even withdraws blood for automatic analysis. These systems regulate delivery only under controlled, well defined treatment procedures, following a set of programmed, precise instructions. These instructions are predetermined by the appropriate medical personnel involved in systems design and development. The computer systems themselves can act in the manner that might be followed by human intervention only after being programmed. Drug administration using infusion pump systems can be considered one type of patient maintenance system.

Holter Monitoring

Ambulatory electrocardiography requires assessment of ECG records by either physicians or technicians. The hours spent in analysis of these records can be costly. The results of the analysis can be adversely affected by the physical status of the personnel making the evaluation. Fatigue of personnel results in marked reduction of accuracy in analysis. Therefore, computerized analysis has been attempted through various methods.

The electrocardiograph analysis is conducted by a **real-time** computer system that reports results in current, up-to-date assessments. Results of the comparisons between the ability of machines and the ability of diagnosticians reflect the ability of the machine to aid significantly in providing diagnostic aid to clinicians. The cost involved in the use of the computer system to analyze electrocardiographs is still quite high. As demand for these systems increase, the costs may decline to a point of cost effectiveness

ISSUES IN THE USE OF AUTOMATED SYSTEMS

The advantages of automated clinical systems revolve around the issues of time of reporting, accuracy and documentation, and reliability and validity. The disadvantages of automated systems must also be considered before automated systems can be developed to overcome the failings of present technology.

Timeliness of Reports. Reporting the results of laboratory and other tests assists providers in making decisions that affect a patient's health status. Perhaps one of the greatest advantages of computerized monitoring systems in the provision of health care results directly from the availability of current, timely reports reflecting the patient's condition.

Documentation and Legibility. Documentation produced by computerized systems tends to be more legible than handwritten notes and observations. More accurate and legible documentation for patient data can result in more appropriate decision making for patient treatment.

Reliability and Validity

Reliability. Reliability is a statistical measurement that reflects the ability to replicate the same results under similar conditions over repeated testing of those conditions. When referring to physiological monitoring systems or other automated types of equipment, the measurement of reliability gives an assessment of the performance of the machine over a period of time with repeated testing of the same or similar conditions. A high degree of reliability reflects a strong ability to perform consistently over a period of time. A low degree of reliability reflects a poor ability to perform with consistent results.

Validity. Validity is also a statistical measurement that reflects a true or accurate state of affairs. When referring to automated medical equipment, validity reflects an assessment of the ability of the equipment to actually assess a true statement of affairs.

Two terms borrowed from the field of epidemiology may be applied to reflect conditions of validity for automated equipment. These terms are **false positive** and **false negative**. False positive test situations reflect a state of affairs where a test has shown a positive result without the condition being tested for actually being present. False positives are basically the equivalent of a false alarm. False negative test situations reflect the state where a test has given a negative result when the condition being tested for is actually present.

The ability of a test to perform under conditions that provide few false positives and few false negatives can reflect the value of that test or measurement for medical personnel. Certainly under the conditions of a false negative where an alarm condition is actually not being recognized, then some type of backup system for the test must be provided.

Problems with computerized monitoring systems. Several problems have been discussed in relation to the use of computerized physiological monitoring and the use of other automated monitoring systems.

Data collection through monitoring systems result in massive amounts of information that must be evaluated. When health care providers are continually bombarded with continuous information flow, a condition known as **data burnout** or **data overload** may occur. The processing of large amounts of information may result in a reduction in the ability of the observer to recognize significant pieces of information.

When data is overlooked or mistakenly evaluated, particularly in an intensive care situation, the result may adversely affect the treatment outcome for a patient. For this reason, computerized systems capable of recognition of significant data are being developed and implemented.

Another problem with output from automated systems frequently cited is that of data redundancy. Data redundancy refers to the possibility that measurements taken may be repetitive and of little clinical value. Development of data that is relevant to patient assessment and treatment must be developed in conjunction with automated systems in order to produce effective systems.

Technical inexperience of staff may also be a problem in the use of automated systems. Particularly in critical care areas, computerized systems have developed at such a rapid rate many professionals find their initial professional training to be insufficient. Technical inexperience may result in measurements being taken that cannot be analyzed appropriately by personnel or in equipment malfunctions that cannot be adequately assessed by personnel. The technical level of expertise required in using equipment may be too high and the level of expertise in available personnel may not meet requirements.

Health care professionals need to interact with the computer industry to enable the design and manufacture of computer equipment that is relevant and useful in the provision of patient care. Measurements collected must be developed carefully to avoid data redundancy, data burnout and data overload. Computerized systems must be developed to increase the ease of operation and proper training of personnel must be provided.

Fault Tolerance

No Fault Tolerance and Zero Down Time. Computer systems that monitor patients in critical care areas or that act as decision support systems involved in patient care need to be reliable in their results and available for use when needed. Most of us have experienced the frustration of dealing with computer "down-time" in one form or another. Down-time may be entirely unacceptable when working with patient data in a critical care environment.

The 1990s buzzword for clinical computing systems may involve the concept of **no fault tolerance**. Basically the concept relies on delivery of a central processing unit capable of being available for use at a rate of 99%. **Zero down-time** is another term that also refers to a high rate of availability of the central processing unit for use when needed. This reliability may be achieved through the use of two processors cooperating within the central processing unit and also through allowing for backup to take place while the computer system is still available for use by clinical staff.

The concept of no fault tolerance however, does not frequently take into account down-time on other parts of the computer system's components besides the central processing unit. Input and output devices are subject to maintenance requirements and may affect the total operating capacity for the system. Reasonable expectations for downtime need to realize the dependence of the entire system upon each of the components that make up that system, including peripherals such as disk drives, monitors, light pens, keyboards, and printers. Backups for these hardware components may need to be considered if a high degree of availability is actually required of a system for use in clinical environments.

CHAPTER SUMMARY

This chapter focuses on computerized applications that have been designed primarily for direct patient care and treatment. These applications include health assessment systems, clinical monitoring systems and special purpose systems. Reliability and validity issues are explored.

Health assessment systems are designed to aid in the determination of a patient's health status. These systems can be either general (providing a screening mechanism), or problem specific (assisting in the recognition of particular categories of disorders).

Clinical monitoring systems and special purpose systems may utilize sensor technology to monitor patients in clinical environments. Systems have been developed and implemented that perform physiological monitoring, arrhythmia monitoring, obstetrical and neonatal monitoring, drug administration, and patient maintenance.

The advantages of automated systems include the timeliness and legibility of reports. Drawbacks of automated systems include the technical inexperience of staff, data burnout, and data redundancy.

TERMINOLOGY AND REVIEW EXERCISES

Essential Vocabulary

general health assessment systems
physiological monitoring systems
arrythmia monitoring systems
pulmonary monitoring systems
obstetrical/neonatal monitoring systems
special purpose systems
sensor
transducer

Essential Vocabulary *(continued)*

signal processing units
automated medical instrumentation
patient bedside management systems
computer-assisted diagnosis
dedicated computer systems
turnkey respiratory function systems
drug administration systems
infusion pumps
Holter monitoring
patient maintenance systems
real-time system
reliability
validity
vaporizers
false positive
false negative
data burnout
data overload
no fault tolerance
zero down time

True/False

1. Health assessment software evaluates patient response to questions that result in an indicator of health status.
2. Dedicated computer systems generally are multipurpose, capable of performing a wide variety of data processing functions.
3. Arrhythmia monitoring systems may perform surveillance functions as well as diagnostic capabilities.
4. Data overload refers to the overdelivery of data for provider evaluation which may impede accurate assessment.
5. Reliability is a statistical measurement which reflects a true or accurate state of affairs.
6. Patient maintenance systems are experimental systems capable of limited diagnostics and treatment under carefully controlled conditions.
7. Transducers are part of signal processing units and alter or filter initial input picked up by the sensing device to make the output easier to read and evaluate.
8. Drug administration systems include vaporizers and infusion pumps.
9. Zero down time may be accomplished through the implementation of appropriate backup procedures.
10. Holter monitoring is a type of patient monitoring for ambulatory cardiology patients.

Fill in the Blanks

1. ____________ ____________ and ____________ ____________ are measurements which reflect the validity of a particular test.
2. A high degree of ____________ reflects a strong ability to perform consistently over a period of time.
3. Modular physiological monitoring systems are frequently called ____________ ____________ ____________ or ____________ ____________ ____________ ____________.

4. ____________________ ____________________ ____________________ refers to the capacity of a computer system to provide diagnostic assistance to health care providers.
5. Obstetrical and neonatal units utilize ____________________ ____________________ ____________________ to monitor patients in these units.
6. One example of a ____________________ ____________________ computer system is a drug administration system.
7. ____________________ ____________________ are electronic instrumentation capable of detecting minute changes in measurements such as temperature, pressure, or other physiological measurements.
8. Feedback control mechanisms for signal processing units can be either ____________________ or ____________________ ____________________ systems.
9. ____________________ ____________________ ____________________ ____________________ provide complete total pulmonary function analysis.

Review Questions

1. List and describe the types of clinical monitoring systems currently in use in critical care areas.
2. Discuss the issues of the reliability and validity of computer systems in clinical settings.
3. Discuss the advantages and disadvantages of health assessment computer systems.
4. Identify and discuss the issues in the use of computerized systems in clinical monitoring systems.

Chapter 11

Artificial Intelligence and Expert Systems

Chapter Outline

OBJECTIVES
ARTIFICIAL INTELLIGENCE
DEFINITIONS OF ARTIFICIAL INTELLIGENCE
PHILOSOPHICAL CONSIDERATIONS IN THE AREA OF ARTIFICIAL INTELLIGENCE
ARTIFICIAL INTELLIGENCE METHODOLOGIES
CHALLENGES FOR RESEARCHERS IN ARTIFICIAL INTELLIGENCE
ROBOTICS
EXPERT SYSTEMS IN HEALTH CARE
CHAPTER SUMMARY
TERMINOLOGY AND REVIEW EXERCISES

OBJECTIVES

1. Define artificial intelligence.
2. Discuss the philosophical considerations of artificial intelligence research.
3. Define and discuss searching techniques used in the production of artificial intelligence systems.
4. Discuss the development of robotics and its current applications in health care.
5. Discuss some of the challenges being faced today by AI researchers.
6. Explore the use of expert systems in health care.
7. Describe some of the current expert systems being used as decision support systems in health care.
8. Present some of the social and legal implications of using expert systems in the field of medicine.

ARTIFICIAL INTELLIGENCE

Artificial intelligence is certainly one of the most fascinating areas of study that has developed as a direct consequence of the breakthroughs in computer technology. The questions that researchers are studying in this area are varied and complex, ranging from achieving computerized sensory input and perception, to playing chess games, pitting the computer against champions who play at the grand master level. The challenges being met in this field make it one which holds rich promise for current and future advancements in medical diagnosis and treatment.

The Turing Test

Alan M. Turing, a scientist in the 1950s, introduced the provocative question of whether or not machines were capable of thought. In addition, he proposed an objective method for determination of the presence of the "intelligent" ability—his method is now known as the **Turing test**. The test involves the discrimination of an interrogator (A) in response to interactions with another individual and a machine (B and C). Communication occurs through a terminal allowing for no visual contact. The basic requirement is that the interrogator (A) be able to ascertain through questioning the machine and the human which (either B or C) is actually the machine. If (A) is not able to discriminate between the human and the computer, beyond what is expected by chance, then the machine can be said to display human intelligence.

Even though many years have passed since the development of the Turing Test, it is still considered a means for measuring the "intelligence" of a machine. Researchers believe that eventually computers will pass the Turing Test.

DEFINITIONS OF ARTIFICIAL INTELLIGENCE

Artificial intelligence (AI) has been viewed until recently as a branch of computer science that worked on practical applications based on developments within other fields of science. The research objectives of artificial intelligence have remained so broad that there is no one universally accepted definition of what it entails.

Researchers have examined areas of perception, decision-making, general problem solving, what constitutes "common sense," language and linguistics, and cybernetics. The common thread that links these varied approaches of study is the objective of developing artificial or electronic/mechanical means of accomplishing tasks that were previously accomplished only by human beings.

Artificial intelligence, therefore, may be defined as an applied science involved in the study and development of technology that possesses a demonstrable ability to imitate the characteristics of human processes such as perception, movement, intuition, communication, and decision-making.

This definition is sufficiently broad to include the various fields of inquiry currently exploring artificial intelligence developments. At the same time, the definition purposely uses the term "imitate" to imply an inherent difference between machine intelligence and capabilities and that of human intelligence and achievements. While recognizing that the term imitate differentiates between the machine and the human, the lines which mark the difference between human intelligence and machine intelligence may, sometime in the future, become indistinguishable. Perhaps, in some instances, machine intelligence may even surpass present human capacities.

PHILOSOPHICAL CONSIDERATIONS IN THE AREA OF ARTIFICIAL INTELLIGENCE

Human beings are capable of conscious thought. This fact appears to us, most of the time, self evident. However the dimensions of the terms consciousness and thought become somewhat hazy when we begin to study artificial intelligence.

Of course the ability to choose between two alternatives constitutes a decision. Does having the ability to make a decision constitute thought? Is there any consciousness inherent in the ability to make a choice? If a computer can be programmed to make a choice based upon available data, then does this imply that a computer can think? Does it not imply some rudimentary sense of consciousness? Is not the ability to think and chose purely a human characteristic? If we can program computers to indeed think, then are we not giving to machines that very quality which makes us unique, which makes us human?

What about consciousness? It is defined as the state of being characterized by sensation, emotion, volition, and thought. The term conscious implies an awareness of an "inward state or outward fact." We can program a computer to input data on a perceptual level—for example to understand a human voice and respond to it. Are we not developing the computer to possess some degree of consciousness? Are there levels of consciousness that have previously been unrecognized?

If we are, in fact, sharing the characteristics which make us human with computer systems, then what meaning will this have for our future? What are the implications in terms of how we have understood our very nature?

These are the types of questions that the field of artificial intelligence has thrust upon us. Philosophers and scientists ponder questions about the very substance of our species with a vigor that has not been witnessed for quite some time.

Other questions have evolved concerning the utilization of artificial intelligence systems. Proponents of artificial intelligence recognize that computer systems are capable of producing consistent and reliable results; these results are generally achieved at a speed and degree of reliability that sometimes cannot be matched by humans.

While computers may not be able, at this point in time, to perceive or assess the complexities involved in decision making, proponents realize these computer systems can be put to good use in areas previously thought to be the exclusive domain of human beings.

Many reports have cited the dangers inherent in allowing machines control over life-threatening situations. Weapons control and the possible computer error involved in machine control have frequently been mentioned as one of the "scary" possibilities brought about through the use of artificial intelligence systems.

End-of-the-world scenarios are discussed as possibilities brought about by "high tech" weapons systems, their development aided, in part, by research completed in artificial intelligence laboratories. Many scientists have voiced their fears that perhaps there are areas of study which should be abandoned, based solely on the potential for harm.

As with most developments of technology, the uses that can be made of artificial intelligence depend largely upon the intent of the user. The destructive capability of a machine is largely dependent upon human intention. While great sums of money are being spent to develop weapons systems, and their benefits to mankind remain the subject of much debate, expenditures in AI development within the medical industry show the wide range of benefits that this technology can bring to mankind.

ARTIFICIAL INTELLIGENCE METHODOLOGIES

Initial explorers in the realms of artificial intelligence began with a relatively simple challenge—trying to teach a computer how to play games—checkers, backgammon, and chess being some of the most common. Early researchers, through the effort of trying to program the computer with the basic instructions necessary to play the game, began to identify and understand some fundamental concepts involved in decision making.

Two concepts that continue to play important functions in AI research were outlined, **searching techniques** and **knowledge representation**.

Searching and Heuristics

Searching is a technique developed in AI that examines problem states, defined as successive and alternative stages in the problem solving process. An example of a problem state would include the configuration of a chess board before the opening move, along with all possible moves and results of those moves that could be made by the game pieces on the board at that time. In order for any reasonable, nonrandom choice (whether human or machine) to be made, searches must be made of a problem state and some of the alternatives explored. The number of alternatives, depending on the number of moves that can be made, and the possible outcomes based upon those moves, makes searching in some games extremely complex.

The average number of moves in a chess game at any one time is 35. Looking ahead only 3 moves has been estimated to require examination of 1.8 billion moves. The large number of possibilities and alternatives represent what is known as a **combinatoral explosion** and makes the development of a program capable of assimilating all information extremely difficult. Computer programs are therefore organized in their methods of searching to simplify the possibilities that must be considered before a decision is reached.

Because of the numbers of alternatives involved in playing even a simple game, AI researchers developed search procedures that would aid in problem-solving. Many AI investigators believe that humans often employ search procedures to aid them in problem solving, and that searching abilities are fundamental to what we term intelligent behavior.

A mechanism for simplifying the alternatives to be considered must be available. The mechanisms for simplifying choices and guiding the direction of a decision making process are termed **heuristics**. They are rules of thumb or problem solving strategies that may be followed. There is no guarantee, however, when a heuristic technique is implemented that it will result in a correct or winning choice.

Nevertheless, scientists believe that heuristics play an important role in guiding human choices and limiting the number of choices from which humans ultimately make a choice. Research in heuristic techniques is an ongoing effort and will continue as a legitimate field of inquiry for AI researchers indefinitely. One of the benefits of heuristic research is the insight it has leant into the boundaries of effective decision making.

Knowledge Representation

Knowledge representation requires that all relevant information about a particular problem area be collected. Along with the ability to describe that information and its interrelationships, this initial collection of data must be described in an appropriate computer language.

Knowledge representation for playing a chess game would have to include a description of the board, the pieces, the moves each piece is capable of making and, of course, the purpose of the game. Relationships between pieces would have to be established—such as the relative values of each game piece. All information must be programmed in an appropriate computer language before knowledge representation is accomplished.

Production rules are one method of knowledge representation where the system is defined by a set of rules based on what is known as an **IF . . . THEN structure**. Rule based systems or production systems consist of the complete set of production rules that govern a particular application. Each production rule contains information that can be inserted or deleted from the total system so that it is possible to update the system as needed. If the system is a complex one, it may be necessary to break the production rules into subsets that make problem management and maintenance of the system somewhat easier. Expert systems that aid in medical diagnosis lend themselves to knowledge representation in this format. A review of some current expert systems used in heath care facilities will be covered later in this chapter.

Expert systems are all basically composed of 1) knowledge representation in the form of rules and 2) a computer program that can interpret and act on these rules. The rules are known as the **knowledge base** and the program is called the **inference or reasoning engine**. The IF section is often termed the antecedent or condition whereas the THEN section is the action or consequence. Basically, any program that tests for conditions and then takes action on the basis of the result of the testing can be called a **rule based system.**

Statistical Pattern Recognition

Statistical pattern recognition is another frequently employed methodology within the study of artificial intelligence, particularly in the development of expert systems for diagnosis. Statistical pattern recognition (SPR) actually defines a problem area, develops lists of possible features that could be present, and relates them in a probabilistic manner to possible disease categories. Consult-I is an example of an expert system that employs this method.

There are many other methodological systems in artificial intelligence research that are being explored for their usefulness. It is beyond the scope of this text to define and discuss all of them. However, this area of inquiry offers tremendous hope for the future advancement of health care technology and delivery.

CHALLENGES IN STUDY OF ARTIFICIAL INTELLIGENCE

Investigating the ability to program computers to process language is one of the greatest challenges researchers face in developing artificial intelligence. It is a fascinating journey into the complexities of human communications and the subtleties involved in human intellect.

Conveying meaning is one of the purposes of communication. When humans communicate, they are capable of conveying meaning in many ways, through facial expressions, tone of voice, or in the context of what has previously been stated or understood.

When programming computers to respond on the basis of words, it can be quite difficult to account for differences in contextually based meanings. Take for example the simple phrase "May Day!" The phrase may be written on a banner strung between two trees in a park with the intent of announcing the location of the annual spring festival. The sign will probably evoke feelings of pleasure and gaiety—a sense associated with a nice gathering on a clear spring day. If the same term is received over Coast Guard airways, then the meaning "May Day!" has changed dramatically as does the response. Concern develops rapidly as Coast Guard personnel attempt to locate a ship or plane that may be in serious trouble. The *context* of language is a powerful influence of the ability to understand the meaning.

Another phrase that conveys ambiguity might be "Important Patients Sign Up Here." This particular phrase might be frequently seen in many reception areas in medical clinics. To most humans the meaning is clear because of context of the situation. The sign conveys to us the importance of signing in when we enter the clinic so that we may be seen by our doctor as soon as possible. However, to a computer, the statement might convey an additional meaning—and the computer might be incapable of discerning just who the important patients are who must sign up.

Disambiguating is the term AI researchers use to convey the problem of communicating to a computer system in order to enable the system to distinguish ambiguous factors. Since computers do not perceive context as humans are capable of doing, rules must be defined so that computers can make appropriate responses under particular conditions.

ROBOTICS

The development of robotics technology is closely woven to artificial intelligence development. **Robotics** is one of the challenging areas of study in artificial intelligence research.

Factories currently employ robotic technology. These manufactured friends have successfully assumed job responsibilities that are dangerous and hazardous to man. Examples include working with toxic chemicals or performing problematic industrial tasks. Robots have also been developed to take over the dull, repetitive tasks of the assembly line and each year more robots are working at these tasks.

Social scientists predict that there will continue to be increases in robotic employment as the cost of robotics declines and labor costs continue to increase. Today robots can spray paint automobiles, lift heavy objects, weld heavy metals, and perform routine tasks. The movements of the industrial robot are controlled through a microprocessor and generally the robot is programmed to perform simple operations repeatedly. The robot's actions must be monitored so that correction can occur if necessary.

Other robot technology is developing that combines artificial intelligence technology such as machine vision, touch, and movement with problem solving abilities. These robots are capable of more complex skills with their movements programmed toward goal achievement. Within a manufacturing environment, increased production is frequently the result of robotic efforts.

Robotic sensory perception is generally achieved through the use of TV cameras that "read" or "see" data from the environment and transfer this data into information processed by the robotic brain, its computer. Appropriate responses are then chosen and acted upon.

SHAKEY was the first robot capable of moving across the room by visualizing its environment. It made choices and decisions that enabled it to move across the room unhindered by obstacles placed within its path.

SHAKEY's computer devised a map of the room and the placement of the obstacles. Obstacles were evaluated by their ability to actually block SHAKEY's ability to move across the room. After this processing had been completed, SHAKEY was ready for his first movement.

Once the first step was taken, then the process of evaluation was repeated. SHAKEY used a number of microprocessors for this journey, some controlling motion, some vision, and, of course, overall control of function.

Robotic sensory perception has progressed to a degree where industrial robots use cameras to locate objects and guide assembly operations in limited perceptual fields. Many scientists believe that the generalized ability of computer visual perception is a major key to breakthroughs in artificial intelligence systems. These scientists pursue developments that will allow computers to define their visual environments and actually learn from them. This pursuit continues to challenge researchers.

Meanwhile, developments are occurring in areas where computers actually perform above human potential. These areas include picture processing and image enhancement. Examples of applications using these technologies that have been developed in the health care industry include karotyping chromosomes and counting blood cells.

Robotic technology has also generated development of computer based artificial limbs technology. Amputees are participating in research studies for the development of electronically controlled prostheses. Patients who lack muscular control are also being worked with to develop computer operated devices that will allow the patients musculoskeletal movement and control. These areas of research, mainly derived from robotics development, offer exciting possibilities for the handicapped, paralyzed, and disabled.

EXPERT SYSTEMS IN HEALTH CARE

The State of the Art

The development of the diagnostic tools called **expert systems** is leading to interesting developments in understanding basic diagnostic and clinical reasoning, elucidating and clarifying the processes by which clinical judgments are made.

Expert systems within the medical field have a wide range of applications. They are being used in clinical decision making. In this particular application they may be referred to as **decision support systems**. This terminology tends to reflect the idea that expert systems are not being developed with the idea of replacing human physicians with computers but rather they are being developed in order to facilitate and enhance clinical judgment. The terminology may aid the acceptance of computer aided diagnostics. The term originated in financial management software and was used to express the idea that software could act to aid in decision-making.

One advantage of an expert system is that it puts the knowledge of top specialists to use by less experienced physicians, allowing them to help patients, to improve their treatments, and learn during the process. Expert systems can free the already busy specialist to concentrate on challenging cases. Further, knowledge from experts can be retained and updated.

Examples of Current Applications

MYCIN is a diagnostic computer system that aids in the diagnosis and treatment of bacterial infections of the blood and of the cerebro-spinal (meningeal) fluid. MYCIN utilizes production rule formats and is programmed with the programming language, LISP, that translates the rules into an easy-to-understand English format. MYCIN was developed at Stanford University in the 1970s.

MYCIN first "questions" the user of the system, acquiring the information necessary to search through the many rules in order to properly identify the "correct" choice; it prints that choice in the IF THEN statement giving the probability of that choice being the correct one. Only when the probability coefficient is 1.0 is there complete confidence in the conclusions MYCIN has drawn. To date, MYCIN has been used in research into knowledge representation and has performed a teaching role for medical students. Software known as EMYCIN has been developed for use in designing expert systems based on the principles used to develop MYCIN. Other auxiliary software tools include GUIDON which facilitates the use of MYCIN as a teaching tool.

An example of a MYCIN production rule follows:

IF

1. the infection is primarily bacteremia, and
2. the site of the culture is one of the sterile sites, and
3. the suspected portal of entry of the organism is the gastrointestinal tract,

THEN
there is suggestive evidence (.7) that the identity of the organism is bacteroides.

Note the IF . . . THEN structure of the production rule.

An incredible amount of time was spent in the development of MYCIN. Almost twenty man years were involved in the completion of MYCIN program. Now knowledge based systems can require one to five man years to complete. It is due to the pioneering efforts of the beginning artificial intelligence scientists that this reduction in time and resources is now possible.

MYCIN, of course, has been tested for the validity of its results in comparison to human specialists. In one comparison, MYCIN tests at 65% where the range of correct choices from the human specialists was 42.5–62.5% of cases tested. This type of analysis reflects the validity of the MYCIN program as a decision support system.

Although expert systems initially focus on diagnostics within a limited problem domain, the abilities to expand systems is becoming feasible. **INTERNIST/CADUCEUS** is a system developed initially by Harry Pople and others at the University of Pittsburgh.

QMR or **Quick Medical Reference** has built upon the knowledge base of INTERNIST. Disease profiles have been set up for 591 internal medicine classifications. The system will eventually contain approximately 750 disease profiles. An AT system with a 286 microprocessor is needed to run the QMR system on an IBM compatible computer with 512K Random Access Memory. A hard disk is also required. The QMR program has several features that permit viewing the disease profile itself, as well as providing ranked listings of probable diagnoses for a particular set of patient symptoms. It is also capable of suggesting testing protocols for differential diagnostics based on those tests that are the least expensive to perform and/or the least invasive (risky) for the patient.

Different levels of information provided with the QMR system allow for use of the program in multiple roles. It is a diagnostic tool. QMR can complete a full diagnostic analysis in 1 to 4 hours depending on factors involved in each particular case. Disease profiles can be called up in less than a minute. QMR can also be used as an information tool for patient care and education.

Evaluation of the QMR system is still underway but initial results reflect positive trends including diagnostic sensitivity equivalent comparable to a consulting physician and consistently better than that of less experienced ward diagnostic teams. QMR is also viewed by the clinicians using it as educationally helpful.

Social and Legal Issues

Expert systems aiding in diagnosis are a reality. As research and technology continue to develop, changes in the provision of health care will surely ensue. Social and legal questions will arise that cannot be answered now but will certainly be of major interest to our society in the coming years.

Some of the questions include:

- Will doctors and physicians continue to administer care for day-to-day illnesses and common aches and pains or will their role become one of a supervisory nature?
- Will patients demand computer aided diagnoses?
- Will this practice become a new standard of care?

These questions reflect the changing nature of the delivery of medical and health services. Computer systems are playing a radical role in transforming the delivery system and can be expected to continue to impact upon delivery of services in the future.

Liability issues will occur from errors in diagnosis. Will manufacturers of medical expert systems be held liable for these misdiagnoses? What will the extent of that liability be? Can the physician experts who contribute to the development of expert systems also be held liable in medical malpractice suits and, if so, what will be the extent of *their* liability? Further, what impact will liability have on commercial development of expert systems? What impact will liability have on physician acceptance of the use of computerized diagnostic systems? Will we ever reach the point in time where non-use of computer systems may end up resulting in physician liability if computer systems evolve to consistently offer reliable assessments? If this occurs, what impact will computer diagnostic systems have on the cost of health care services?

These questions and issues remain to be developed and examined as the increasing interfacing between computers and diagnostics continues. The questions are limitless and the answers will certainly be difficult to establish.

Advantages and Limitations of Expert Systems

Expert systems are not capable of replacing medical decision making by the physician. Expert systems are useful in that they provide information that aids the physician in making sound, informed judgments as to the validity of diagnosis and choices for therapy. Because of this ability to aid in the medical decision making process, they have sometimes been called **ancillary consultation devices**. The advantages and limitations of expert systems have not truly been determined at this stage of their development although some observations have been noted.

Limitations of expert systems include the costly requirements of the hardware and software with which to operate an expert system. Another limitation frequently mentioned is the requirements for extensive training in order for medical personnel to become well versed in the use of the system itself.

However it is still too early to evaluate the impact that expert systems will have upon the provision of medical care in the future. As their study and development continues, the true advantages of this technology will be determined.

CHAPTER SUMMARY

The study of artificial intelligence promises to provide exceptional benefits in the health care field. Applications being developed aid visually impaired and hearing impaired individuals. Robotics manufacturers are developing systems that can aid the physically impaired. Artificial intelligence covers many fields of inquiry including language and thought, sensory perception, communication, and decision making.

Expert systems are one result of the intense research being conducted in artificial intelligence. Applying decision-making strategies to fields of knowledge, it has become possible to structure computer programs that imitate the decision-making behaviors of humans. Expert systems are currently being used experimentally to assist in the diagnostic process.

TERMINOLOGY AND REVIEW EXERCISES

Essential Vocabulary

artificial intelligence
Turing test
searching techniques
knowledge representation
combinatoral explosion
heuristics
production rules
IF . . . THEN structure

Essential Vocabulary *(continued)*

knowledge base
inference engine
rule based systems
statistical pattern recognition
disambiguating
robotics
expert systems
decision support systems
MYCIN
INTERNIST/CADUCEUS
Quick Medical Reference
ancillary consultation devices

True/False

1. MYCIN is an expert system used as a decision support system for the diagnosis, treatment, and management of cancer.
2. Robotics in health care today offer advances in aiding the physically disabled.
3. Heuristics is a term used to describe rules of thumb used in simplifying complex decision making.
4. Rule based expert systems generally rely on an IF . . . THEN structure that tests for the presence of conditions and then "decides" based on the results of the testing.
5. A combinatorial explosion refers to the rapid expansion of possible alternatives that may be generated even in such simple situations such as game playing.
6. The legal status of expert systems in terms of product liability has been determined in a landmark Supreme Court decision.
7. QMR is an expert system capable of completing a fully diagnostic analysis in one to four hours depending on the complexity of the factors involved.
8. Ancillary consultation devices are equivalent to decision support systems.

Fill in the Blank

1. The ____________ ____________________ is a procedure through which a machine's capacity for intelligence may be determined.
2. ____________________ is a method for removing ambiguous or confusing structures from the human language.
3. ____________________________ is that portion of research engaged in developing electronic/electrical/mechanical means for performing activities once thought to be only within the capacity of human performance.
4. ____________________ ____________________ ____________________ is a computer system that works with disease profiles for over 500 internal medicine classifications.
5. A production rule system usually has an ______ . . . __________ structure.
6. ____________________ ____________________ ____________________ and ____________________ ____________________ ____________________ are other terms frequently employed in the discussion of expert systems.
7. ____________________________ is the expert system that provides a data base of information on treatment programs for cancer patients.

8. ______________________________ is the expert system that provides information to clinicians on bacterial infections of the blood and cerebro-spinal fluid.
9. ________________________ was the first experimental robot that could move across a room and evaluate obstacles that inhibited its movement.

Review Questions

1. Discuss the wide variety of applications that the study of artificial intelligence systems have helped to develop.
2. Discuss the social and legal issues involved in the utilization of expert systems in health care.
3. Describe three expert systems currently in use in health care today.
4. Describe the role heuristics plays in decision making.

Chapter 12

Diagnostics

Chapter Outline

OBJECTIVES

1. Introduce basic terminology applicable to biomedical imaging processing techniques.
2. Discuss the transmission of analog measurements to digital form for the purpose of graphical representation.
3. Define and describe several computerized diagnostic techniques including computerized tomography, magnetic resonance imaging, and ultrasound imaging.
4. Introduce emerging technology such as optical fibers and laser beams in diagnosis and treatment.

Technological innovation has produced startling new fields of research and inquiry in medical science and health care diagnosis, treatment, and delivery. One of the areas undergoing tremendous development is that of **biomedical image processing**.

The field of study known as biomedical image processing may refer to technical aspects of signal detection and measurement, image production and enhancement, and/or the diagnostic procedures used in the evaluation of the image itself. Biomedical image processing employs a variety of technological innovations in the production of images for biomedical purposes. **Diagnostic or clinical imaging** utilizes biomedical images for the purpose of diagnosis, evaluation, and/or treatment. Computerized tomography, radiography, ultrasound, nuclear medicine, and thermography, as well as other biomedical image processing modalities all employ computerized diagnostic imaging techniques. These diagnostic imaging techniques are all based on digital image processing.

The technology involved in the production of digital images is quite complex and beyond the scope of this text. However, a broad overview of the techniques involved in the production of digital images and a discussion of the diagnostic imaging techniques currently employed in clinical settings are particularly relevant to the discussion of the use of computers and computer systems in the health care professions.

DIGITAL IMAGING

A **digital image** represents the presentation of a signal as a two-dimensional pattern. The terms biomedical imaging, clinical imaging, and diagnostic imaging are synonymous terms that reflect the use of **images** in diagnostic, clinical, and medical environments. Medical image processing is concerned with the production of images that will provide patient data that could not easily be obtained by visual means. The images that are produced through medical or diagnostic imaging will provide enhancement and clarification to both the diagnostic and treatment process. Ultimately, diagnostic imaging affects the outcomes of patient care in positive ways.

Most physiological signals used to monitor patients are based on continuous rather than discrete data. Analog signals are considered continuous because they continuously change over time and reflect an infinite set of possible measurements. Before digital imaging can occur, analog signals must be digitized (converted to digital form from their original analog signal). After conversion of the original data has taken place, other steps must be taken to produce a clear, useful image. These steps include signal enhancement and data manipulation. Once these steps have taken place, then data can be analyzed and processed to exemplify important data characteristics that serve to aid in diagnosis and treatment.

Basically, all diagnostic imaging methods attempt measurement of tissues and/or internal body structures. Any digital images representing these internal structures are based on a large number of these measurements being taken, then transformed through mathematical manipulations. The mathematical transformation results in the ability to produce an image based on the patient tissue characteristics previously measured.

The use of digital imaging in medical diagnosis provides diagnosticians with an exceptional breakthrough. Perhaps the most important characteristic of diagnostic imaging is that it allows for clinical judgments to be made *without* invasive, exploratory surgical procedures, Figure 12–1.

COMPUTER ASSISTED TOMOGRAPHY

Computerized Tomography (CT) or **Computer Assisted Tomography** (CAT) is a diagnostic tool that allows for the production of digitalized images of organs and tissues after passing the body through a scanning device. X-ray beams pass through the body and construct images from the density of various organs or structures in the body. Soft tissues in the body can be differentiated effectively because the density of an organ's tissue structure will affect

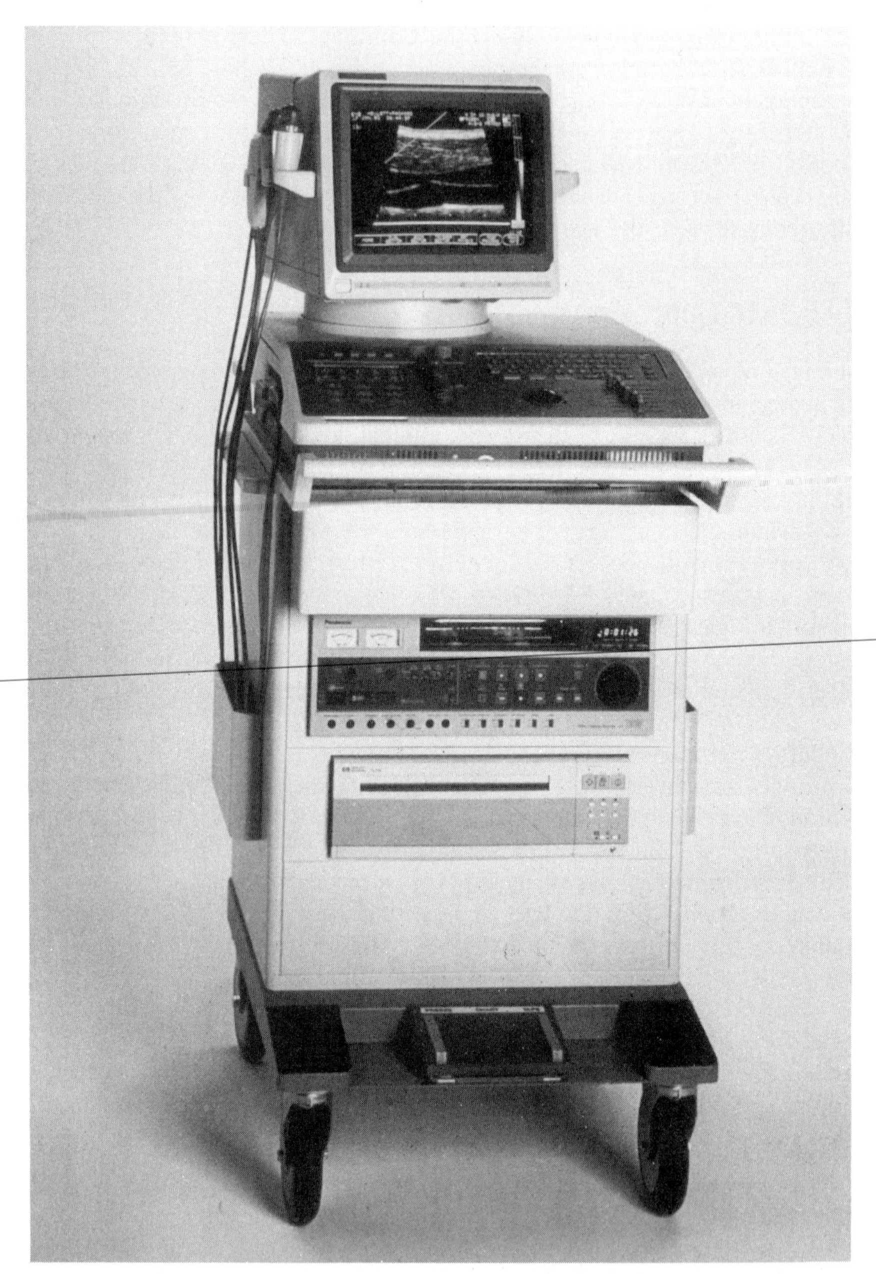

Figure 12–1 The HP SONOS 1000 cardiovascular imaging system from Hewlett-Packard Company (with optional cart and recording devices) is a fully equipped, mobile ultrasound system. The system's size, mobility, price, and high performance features make it an ideal system for the private office, clinic, or mobile service, yet it is powerful enough for the hospital. ***(Courtesy of Hewlett-Packard Company)***

how the X-ray beams are absorbed. The differences in absorption will eventually be reflected in the image that the computer will develop. The computer itself is actually responsible for decoding the raw data and then rebuilding the image following the programmed instructions of the computer system.

Images processed through the computerized tomography systems offer clinicians a more distinguishable form useful in analysis and diagnosis. The term tomography refers to sectioning, and the unique ability of computerized tomography to actually produce a cross sectional representation of a slice of the patient's body is what makes it such a powerful diagnostic tool.

Conventional X-rays can be confusing because the images they produce provide a two-dimensional rather than a three-dimensional representation of the human body. Because CT produces an image that has not been superimposed or, in effect, layered, the image produced can be more precise and discerning.

Computerized tomography was first introduced commercially in 1972. Since that time it has been rapidly implemented as a diagnostic tool in research facilities, hospitals, and other health care facilities. The cost of such a scanning device can reach into the hundreds of thousands of dollars. However, the resulting benefits for a large patient population have been well established.

Computerized tomography has been implemented in a diagnostic capacity in several areas of medicine. The neurosciences employ CT for scanning patients with severe head injuries or with suspected brain tumor growth. Cerebrospinal analysis is also possible using computerized tomography. Many areas previously unaccessible through standard X-rays can now be examined, analyzed, and evaluated through the use of CT technology. CT appears very sensitive to detecting the differences in densities of tissues that conventional methods cannot.

Computerized tomography, since its introduction in the 1970s, has undergone major innovations, including a considerable time reduction in producing a useable digitized image. The image can be reconstructed from as many as one million "samples" of data. The image is achieved with higher resolution and a minimum exposure of radiation for the patient undergoing the scan.

Algorithms are techniques employed to turn the sample measurements taken from the patient by the scanner into a useable form for diagnostic evaluation. One example of a computer tomographic algorithm is the algebraic reconstruction technique. These algorithms guide the formation of the reconstructed image and enable users to modify variables such as resolution and image quality.

MAGNETIC RESONANCE IMAGING

Magnetic Resonance Imaging (MRI) or **Nuclear Magnetic Resonance Imaging** is a relatively new technology that appears to offer much promise. It is based on the measurement of nuclear magnetic resonance signals. A data base is generated from coding the measurement of the density of resonating nuclei along with two relaxation times. Most of the clinical MRI systems focus on the measurement of hydrogen nuclei at the present time.

The images produced can characterize different tissues and has been shown to be particularly effective in distinguishing lesions in the brain and spinal cord. This particular imaging modality is more expensive than that of computerized tomography but the powerful ability of MRI to visualize lesions and other soft internal tissues without resorting to the use of ionizing radiation will insure its continued development and use.

MRI has been demonstrated to be effective in determining the presence of tumors in internal tissues. Machines now exist that are capable of imaging entire body cross sections. MRI is being developed as a diagnostic and treatment tool for the detection of tumors and the monitoring of tumor growth during treatment.

One advantage of magnetic resonance imaging over CT is that MRI allows for exceptional resolution and offers enhanced contrast resolution of soft tissue. Intravenous injection of contrast material is unnecessary because of this capacity of MRI to directly image the spinal cord without administration of contrast material.

MRI has been studied in comparison to CT and shown to be better than CT for brain displays. The modality of MRI appears to be more effective than CT for detection of inflammatory processes, hemorrhage, and edema associated with brain tumors.

One other advantage of MRI is that it frequently can differentiate among tissue structures such as fat, muscle, or blood vessels that may look like similar structures on a CT image. MRI has been effectively utilized in diagnostic imaging of the musculoskeletal system, the abdomen, the heart, and cardiovascular system.

Disadvantages of MRI include contraindications for use with patients that have pacemakers or intracranial aneurysm clips. Patient movement may also lead to imaging problems and one complaint of patients undergoing MRI is that of claustrophobia. Specificity may also be a problem with MRI, however, it should be noted that MRI is still undergoing development and many of these disadvantages may be overcome as the technology develops.

ULTRASOUND IMAGING

When X-rays are not advisable, another imaging system can be utilized. In **ultrasound imaging** the imaging is performed on the basis of measurement of the acoustic properties of tissue. In some instances this particular imaging technique can provide a useful characterization of patient tissues. Ultrasound has been demonstrated to be effective in obstetrics for measuring fetal development in the uterus. Cardiology has applied ultrasound technology for imaging of the heart. Ultrasound can aid in distinguishing between soft tissues that may not be successfully represented by computed tomography systems.

The main advantage of the use of ultrasound as a diagnostic imaging technique is in its safety. It has proved to be an excellent choice when there exists any potential danger from the use of radiation. Ultrasound produces no known adverse affects when used for diagnostic procedures. One disadvantage exists when using ultrasound for postoperative evaluations. Dressings, retention sutures, and open wounds produce difficulties in performing ultrasound procedures.

One of the most exciting properties of ultrasound technology is its ability to provide a visual impression of an organ in motion. In combination with the advantage of protecting the patient from possibly harmful effects of radiation through the use of X-ray or radioactive tracers, ultrasound technology is finding a wide spread acceptance in clinical application. Researchers are applying ultrasound technology in new ways and are developing methods of **ultrasound tomography**, with the use of ultrasound instead of X-ray.

Advanced ultrasound imaging technology allows for digital imaging to be applied to moving tissue. One method is that of **gated ultrasoundography.** This method is used to generate images of rhythmically moving tissues or muscles, such as found in the heart.

Another advanced method being developed using ultrasound technology is the **pulsed or gated Doppler imaging**. This particular method has been applied to image erythrocytes moving in blood vessels, allowing for visualization of the vascular system.

Ultrasound tomography and other advanced ultrasound imaging systems use algorithms to provide the reconstruction of data to produce a visual representation of what is occurring in the patient or the tissue being visualized.

EXPANDING TECHNOLOGIES AND RESEARCH

Fiber Optics and Lasers: The New Treatment Tools

Developments within the computer industry surrounding the use of **fiber optics** as a communications media has led to some correspondingly fascinating developments within the medical community in applying fiber optics to diagnostic and treatment problems. Technology continues to expand diagnostic and treatment potentials for noninvasive medical procedures.

Optical fibers are clear glass fiber strands each of which have the approximate thickness of a strand of human hair. Using a laser device it is possible to use a fiber optic cable to transmit information at amazing speed. A fiber optic cable has ten times the data transmission capacity as a standard coaxial cable. A further advantage of fiber optic cable is that it is very lightweight and also flexible.

Physicians are now using fiber optic cable to literally take a look inside the body. It is possible to view the lungs, inside the intestine, and even the human heart chambers. Fiber optic sensors are being developed that can perform blood analysis at the bedside. In addition, fiber optics in conjunction with laser technology are being used to perform medical procedures that once required invasive surgery. This technology can be expected to increase its impact on the delivery of medical and health care well into the next decade.

The diagnostic device utilizing optical fibers, the **fiberscope**, was first developed at the University of Michigan School of Medicine in 1957 in order to view the stomach and esophagus. From that initial development fiberscopes have developed to allow for the viewing of literally every internal organ. Generally fiberscopes consist of two bundles of optical fibers, one termed an illuminating bundle and the other, the imaging bundle. The **illuminating bundle** transmits light to the human tissue to be observed and the **imaging bundle** is responsible for transmitting the image to an output device for viewing and analysis.

Endoscopes are generally used to view internal organs and tissue. These devices incorporate the fiberscope technology and provide additional channels through which to perform a variety of functions. Water and air can be channeled or fluids can be drained in order to improve visibility. Other channels may provide mechanisms for directing the tip of the endoscope or for providing tiny cutting tools to be used in surgical procedures. Still other channels may provide a pathway for the injection of pharmacological substances.

Fiberscope technology provides innumerable benefits. In general, fiberscopes are proving to be a cost effective technology for providing laboratory analysis with fiber optic sensors. Fiber optic sensors are generally safe and capable of sensitive detection. Fiber optic devices are currently available commercially and are still in the early stages of research and development.

Some of the applications still under experimental development include the use of optic fiber technology to detect and treat tumors. Fluorescence endoscopy is used to detect lung tumors that may be too small for detection by computer assisted tomography or by x-ray. A therapy called photodynamic therapy is utilized to selectively destroy the cancer cells based on the differential absorption of a dye that has been injected into the patient. Photochemical reactions are responsible for the destruction of the malignant cells.

Laser angioplasty is another new technique that employs optical fiber and laser technology. This technique is responsible for the removal of obstructions in coronary arteries caused by the buildup of plague on the arterial wall. A **laser endoscope** may be the tool of choice employed in the future that performs the removal of arteriosclerotic plaque.

CHAPTER SUMMARY

This chapter explores computer systems that use biomedical image processing to aid in the diagnostic process. Biomedical image processing is also referred to as diagnostic or clinical imaging. These imaging systems include computerized tomography, radiology, ultrasound, nuclear medicine and thermography. These systems attempt to measure and assess internal body structures and tissues, without exploratory surgery.

These systems represent some of the more innovative and potentially significant medical advances in recent years. Another area that is receiving attention in the research community is that of fiber optics and laser technology. This technology has been applied in communications systems and is now being applied to the health care field.

TERMINOLOGY AND REVIEW EXERCISES

Essential Vocabulary

biomedical image processing
diagnostic or clinical imaging
digital imaging
image
computer assisted tomography
magnetic resonance imaging
nuclear magnetic resonance imaging
ultrasound imaging
ultrasound tomography
gated ultrasoundography
pulsed or gated Doppler imaging
fiber optics
fiberscope
illuminating bundle
imaging bundle
endoscopes
laser endoscopes

True/False

1. Ultrasound endoscopes may be the tool of choice employed to perform the removal of arteriosclerotic plaque in the near future.

2. Computer assisted tomography is often used in patients where ionizing radiation may be contraindicated.
3. Fiberscope technology is an expensive technology and has not yet been determined to be a cost effective approach for providing laboratory analysis.
4. Endoscopes can be used to view internal organs and tissues.
5. In a fiberscope, the imaging bundle is responsible for transmitting light to the human tissue to be observed.
6. Images are generally represented in a three dimensional pattern.
7. Three terms that are basically synonymous are biomedical imaging, clinical imaging, and diagnostic imaging.

Fill in the Blanks

1. ______________ ______________ is a technique responsible for the removal of obstructions in coronary arteries.
2. ______________ ______________ is used to detect lung tumors that may be too small for detection by computer assisted tomography.
3. ______________ are devices that incorporate the fiberscope technology and provide additional channels through which to perform a variety of functions, including channeling water and air, or removal of fluids.
4. ______________ ______________ ______________ refers to the technical aspects of signal detection and measurement, image production and enhancement, and/or the diagnostic procedures used in the evaluation of the image itself.
5. ______________ or ______________ ______________ employs the use of biomedical images for the purpose of diagnosis, evaluation, and/or treatment.
6. ______________ an image refers to the conversion of analog signals to a digital form.
7. ______________ ______________ ______________ allows for the production of digitalized images of organs and tissues after passing the body through a scanning device.
8. ______________ ______________ ______________ allows for exceptional resolution and offers enhanced contrast resolution of soft tissue.
9. ______________ and ______________ ______________ are becoming increasingly important as new emerging technologies utilized in both treatment and diagnostics.

Review Questions

1. Discuss the advantages and limitations of computer assisted tomography as a biomedical imaging device.

2. Discuss the advantages and limitations of nuclear magnetic resonance imaging. Does it have any advantages over computer assisted tomography?
3. Discuss the advantages and limitations of ultrasound imaging.
4. Discuss the development of the use of laser and fiber optic technologies as imaging and diagnostic tools.

Chapter 13

Confidentiality and Patient Rights

Chapter Outline

OBJECTIVES

1. Describe types and methods of computer crimes.
2. Discuss the possible impact of computer crime on medical environments.
3. Describe methods and means of safeguarding organizations from computer crimes.
4. Introduce the American Medical Association guidelines for electronic data processing.
5. Discuss the problems and issues involved in the electronic processing of patient data.
6. Introduce the legal statutes that protect an individual's privacy.
7. Discuss patients' rights in the context of the right to privacy.
8. Define and discuss the terms depersonalization and dehumanization in the context of electronic processing of patient information.

COMPUTER CRIME

When most of us consider the topic of crime we bring to mind images of uniformed police officers, riding in their patrol cars, ready and willing to disarm and arrest burglars or robbers running from the scene of a crime. While we realize these images may be somewhat fanciful, we rarely take the time to reflect on how crime actually occurs in our society. The who, what, where, and how of criminal actions always seem to take us by surprise when we read the headlines of someone in our community being arrested and brought up to face criminal charges. Our frequent response may be one of surprise and bewilderment when we are confronted with how close to home the criminals may be.

Computer crime is frequently startling and amazing; computer crime involves a multitude of crimes being committed with the use and aid of electronic equipment. Computer crime can include the relatively harmless pranks of technologically advanced teenagers as well as the more serious infractions of adults committing felonies such as theft or fraud.

Types of Computer Crime

Many computer crimes occur involving computer equipment, hardware, or software. Thefts of computer equipment can occur in large companies by the employees that work there. Thefts of this type may be quite obvious, involving stolen CPUs or missing monitors. Other thefts might not be quite as easy to detect. Thefts occur when employees make unauthorized copies of software to take home for their individual use. Depending on the cost of the software, these thefts may be considered quite serious offenses in a court of law.

Other computer crimes work through the computer hardware and software to actually commit the offense. Programmers may access savings accounts in banks or other financial institutions and transfer funds to other accounts. Dummy corporations may be set up and invoices sent by the corporation to bill for services never received. The variations on these themes can be endless and sometimes quite difficult to detect.

Software piracy involves the infringement of copyright laws. **Bootleg software** is a term that refers to software that has been gained through unauthorized copying of a computer program. It may involve outright theft through the copying of software programs belonging to someone else. It may involve the use of software by organizations in a means that is directly in conflict with the licensing agreement implied when a purchase of software is made. In order to avoid complications for organizations that use prepackaged software, company policies need to be established that protect the organization from accusations of infringement of copyright laws. Individual employees need to be trained appropriately in order to respect these company policies.

Organizations can and have been held accountable for the actions of their employees when illegal copies of software are being utilized in the daily conduct of business. Civil suits involving large sums of money may be brought against an organization that is allowing unauthorized use of software. Multiple copies of software may be allowed when a **site license** is bought for a particular software package. This license will allow for users to make a limited number of copies of the software for use by the organization at a particular location.

Computer hackers are individuals who make unauthorized entry into computer systems and data banks. Computer hackers have been described frequently as basically harmless, curious individuals who because of their inordinate curiosity have been driven to access information.

The information these hackers access may vary from protected government files to files from information services who normally charge a fee for accessing data. Normally, little damage is done by the hacker. The thrill or payoff for their crime is the knowledge that they have achieved something they were not supposed to have been able to accomplish—access to protected files of information. However, occasionally hackers do damage the files they access and the cost of repairing or replacing damaged files can be very high.

Embezzlement is a frequent computer crime, involving the theft of funds from organizations or businesses. Estimates of computer related embezzlement suggest that undetected embezzlement may reach into the millions of dollars every year. Since computer crimes may not be detected, the estimates are at best guesses of the actual loss being experienced by United States companies and government organizations. These losses may be theft of cash, theft of property, or even theft of services.

Occasionally data will become lost or damaged within an organization. Reasonable and acceptable limits may be established for this type of occurrence within an organization. However, malicious intent may also sometimes enter the situation. When this occurs, then criminal actions may be involved. Disgruntled and unhappy employees sometimes perform these acts assuming a stance of "justified revenge." Some individuals may feel that circumstances provide adequate reason for the destruction or manipulation of data and information. However, individuals within organizations need to be aware that their actions could be construed as criminal destruction of property and that they could be held responsible for their actions in either a civil or criminal court of law.

Time bombs are one of the ways dissatisfied employees "get even." Time bombs are computer programs set up to begin operating at a particular point in time. They may erase important files within a particular data bank, or they may change important data that has been accumulated for business purposes, such as lists of clients, payroll records, or accounts receivable information.

When data is changed with malicious or purposeful intent, it may also be referred to as **data diddling**. Changes that reflect this type of crime may include changes in credit reports and changes in other types of records such as insurance reports, which might benefit the perpetrator in some form or fashion. People who work for organizations and have access to records may "data diddle" and charge for their services.

Another type of embezzlement facilitated through the use of computer programs is **salami shaving**. Salami shaving occurs when a computer program is designed to remove small amounts of money from particular accounts and moves these funds into a private account. This particular type of theft is difficult to track because the sums from each account may be quite small and hard to uncover. When uncovered, they may be assumed to be just a small error of no significance. Added up however, over all accounts and over an extended time frame, considerable sums of money may be embezzled through this particular technique.

Embezzlement or data manipulation cannot occur without access to the computer system. Often **scavenging** techniques are employed to obtain passwords and information on accessing computer systems. Scavenging, gaining information on accessing a particular computer system, is accomplished through searching in trash cans, offices, and hard copy files.

Access to a computer system may occur through other means besides scavenging. **Trap doors** and **trojan horses** are two mechanisms through which unauthorized access may occur. Trap doors are entry mechanisms used by computer programmers to gain access. Trojan horses are concealed programs added by a computer programmer that will allow for authorized access to a particular system. Both these mechanisms require considerable expertise to implement and because of their technical sophistication can be difficult to detect.

Once access to a computer system has been established many types of programs can be inserted into the computer to cause severe problems for the organization. **Computer viruses** are computer programs that have been introduced into the computer system. The viruses are program codes that are sets of instructions designed to achieve a particular task. These viruses may be relatively harmless or they may be designed to erase important files or shut down the computer system completely. Computer viruses are a particular problem for organizations that use communications devices since the virus may originate from outside the organization.

Data leakage may also occur through communication channels. Programmers or others can code confidential information and disguise it. Once the data is disguised it can be removed from an organization for unauthorized purposes.

Computer crime also occurs through **computer data theft** and **computer time theft**. Data theft involves the theft of information from an organization for use in other ways. A typical example of data theft would be that of an employee getting ready to start a competing business removing data files on pricing and product information for use in starting their business.

Computer time theft involves the theft of computer time from an organization. Employees may use computer systems for their own use. Computer supplies such as printing paper may be consumed by employees working on their own projects. When the computer services are used without payment or without permission then theft has occurred.

Wiretapping is also an example of time theft. Communications lines are accessed and the computer system is used without authorization or payment for service. Satellite communication systems are particularly susceptible to wiretapping.

Impact on Medical Environments

The impact of computer crime on health care institutions has not been directly investigated. Rather, certain deductions can be made about the impact of computer crime on medical environments from the types of computer crimes that are occurring in other industries.

Computer crime does occur in medical environments. Any large organization with sophisticated computerized equipment is vulnerable to the types of computer crimes discussed above. While statistics do not exist for the medical industry specifically, isolated documented cases of thefts can be attributed to medical institutions. Vulnerable areas include theft of pharmaceuticals and theft of expensive medical equipment. These types of thefts are facilitated through the use of computers and the manipulation of inventory data.

Many professionals working in a medical environment are not computer programmers and do not possess the technical expertise necessary to track computer crime in their computer systems. Therefore, the medical environment may be more vulnerable to computer crime than other organizations that have large numbers of employees possessing advanced computer science experience.

Appropriate safeguards are required in order to minimize the impact of computer crime on medical environments. Some of these safeguards will be discussed in the following section.

Guarding Against Computer Crime

Safeguards against unethical and illegal accessing and use of computer systems for illegal purposes must be set up for organizations who depend on information systems. Methods must be employed to guard computer systems, computer software, and information.

Safeguarding Information. Protection of information that is contained within the computer system can occur at several levels. Proper storage of secondary storage devices is one method of protecting information. If sensitive information stored on secondary media are adequately stored and access to the storage media adequately protected, then loss, destruction, or manipulation of valuable data may not occur.

Protecting access to information through the use of appropriate security measures such as the use of **passwords** is one method used to protect unauthorized access to computerized data banks. Passwords allow for only people with the proper clearance to be able to access certain systems or sensitive information within the computer system.

Safeguarding Computer Hardware and Software. Physical equipment can be lost, damaged, or stolen. The same is true for software. Software can also be contaminated by program manipulation to cause inestimable damage to both data files and program files.

Educating employees and training them to understand the importance of security measures is one method of insuring minimization of loss and damage to valuable equipment and programs. Informed employees can also follow proper procedures when they have been instructed about computer crime detection and reporting suspicious occurrences within the workplace.

Inventory audits occurring at unscheduled intervals may help guard the organization against equipment loss and theft. Inspections of the computer system itself using surveillance devices for computer viruses may also aid in protecting data and program files.

Safeguarding Against Theft and Embezzlement. Computer crime can occur during regular working hours in front of other workers who are not even aware that a crime is taking place. However, many computer crimes have been detected by monitoring employees who may clock in inordinate amounts of overtime. People having access to the computer may use overtime hours, when large number of employees are not present, for the purpose of constructing their particular method of entering and altering the computer system programs. Restricting access to program files and monitoring those individuals with authorization may protect the organization from serious loss.

ELECTRONIC PROCESSING AND PRIVACY

One of the major concerns in medical environments is the protection of private and confidential medical records. Electronic processing obviously has in a real sense increased the vulnerability of medical and other patient records to invasion by unauthorized individuals.

The confidentiality of patient records is guarded and protected on both ethical and legal grounds. Electronic processing has increased the vulnerability of unauthorized **access** to individual records and therefore, must be considered.

Privacy Legislation

Implemented legislation on the federal level protects information that may be confidential. These laws are designed to protect the individual right to privacy and further to limit access to individual records by organizations or people who might abuse the privilege of access to confidential information.

Several laws protect the rights of the individual with regard to records and records dispersal and storage. These laws include the **Freedom of Information Act of 1970**, **The Privacy Act of 1974**, and **The Education Privacy Act of 1974**. The Freedom of Information Act allows individuals access to data that has been stored about them by the federal government. The Privacy Act states that information stored must have a reasonable purpose and that information collected for one purpose may not be used for any other purpose without the individual's express consent. This act is designed to protect the individual from abuse of information by the federal government. The Education Privacy Act allows individuals access to information about grades and behavioral evaluations made by private and public schools and allows that information to be challenged by the student.

Other more recent legislation protects the individual specifically from data abuses concerning electronic processing. The **Electronic Communications Privacy Act of 1986** has been set up to protect illegal interception of data communications. Other laws have also been enacted that protect individuals from third party access to information in data banks without the individual's knowledge.

These laws are important beginnings for the establishment of standards that will protect the individual from data abuse. However as technology increases medical professionals must be aware of the possibilities of abuse and continue to advocate protection of patient information.

AMA Guidelines for Computer Security

As we have seen, many laws have been enacted to protect the individual from unlawful and unnecessary invasion of private records. Additionally, the American Medical Association has issued guidelines that help to preserve safeguards in the electronic processing of medical or patient data.

Basically, the American Medical Association suggests that standards be adopted and maintained that protect individual, confidential patient information from access by outside sources. These outside sources are external to the health care facility where the patient receives treatment. Any release of database information must be with the informed consent of the patient and the attending physicians. The purpose for the release of information needs to be stated and information use needs to be limited to that initial purpose.

Security measures also are suggested by the AMA, including restriction of access to authorized employees, removal of terminated employees from access to the data processing facilities, appropriate purging of inaccurate data, and security measures for entry to storage facilities that house computerized medical information.

New methods to protect access to data processing facilities or computer data banks may employ **biometric security devices**. These are devices that measure and match some unique aspect of an individual with stored patterns in the computer system's memory. Handprints and fingerprints can be used to facilitate this process or other biometric measures such as voice recognition.

PROTECTION OF THE INDIVIDUAL

While the law protects the individual from disclosure of certain kinds of information and further protects organizations through law from embezzlement or theft, it is frequently the day-to-day procedures that may actually affect data security of an individual's health or medical records.

Medical record security is largely dependent upon the practitioner's respect for the integrity of the medical record. Health professionals are trained to protect the information contained in an individual's medical record. However, the practice of patient confidentiality can frequently fall by the wayside in daily operations. Patients' conditions are discussed over coffee in public restaurants. Individual medical records may be stored in rooms that are accessed by both administrative and nursing staff. Only the constant self-surveillance of vigilant health care professionals can avert the possibly destructive results of unintentional revelation of confidential information.

Medical record security is also facilitated or thwarted by administrative practices which govern medical record access. Protection of facilities from breaking and entering is only a small part of providing data security for medical records. Hospitals frequently allow access to medical records departments without requiring any particular identification procedures. Safeguards for protecting individual data must be implemented which limit access only to personnel with the right to access medical records information.

The problems of maintaining confidentiality of the contents of the medical record become even more problematic when computer systems maintain that data. Clerical workers in medical offices may be working with sensitive data displayed on a terminal screen. Access to this information is available to anyone who happens to walk through the room where the work is taking place.

Data banks frequently contain information that is maintained for the public good. At times these data banks may impair the individual's right to privacy, if not legally then certainly on ethical grounds. Individuals having venereal diseases may have their names and addresses listed in public health department data banks. Confidential records on testing for the HIV virus may be maintained by health clinics and even by insurance carriers. How well these types of records are protected from access and from simple visibility is a reflection on the ability of the health professions to maintain the integrity of the doctor-patient relationship.

Dehumanization and Depersonalization

We are living in the computer age. Hardly any aspect of modern day life is left untouched by the electronic explosion. These machines can in many ways enhance our lives, making our everyday lives more productive and enjoyable. However many aspects of the onset of the technological explosion we are experiencing have lead to questions concerning the quality of the life we live surrounded by computers and increasing automation.

Information is available to everyone and the collection of information has become big business. Marketing strategies are developed and implemented based on information. Consumers are seen as dollar bills to be caught as they pass through the aisles of a store or watch a commercial on television.

Many social scientists have commented on the effects of **dehumanization** and **depersonalization** of our society. All of us have felt to some degree the effects of depersonalization through automation. Our bankers refer to our account numbers rather than our names. Our "number" is called when our food order in a restaurant is processed and ready to serve. What can the effects of automation do to further increase our sense of being "processed"? How will automating aspects of our health care delivery system impact on the increasing aspects of depersonalization in our society?

Because the nature of our work life is changing, more and more jobs will be replaced through automation. How will the health care delivery system be affected by large numbers of displaced and unemployed workers that may be one result of increasing automation? Will these individuals be considered "nonpersons" or will they receive adequate health care? How will the cost of providing health care services to these individuals be covered? What types of services will be available to them? What kind of equality will exist between those who work and those who are incapable of finding employment? How will our values and respect for human life be changed by the increasing changes brought about by technological advance?

The questions that present themselves for discussion are endless and the answers are not obvious or self-evident. The changes in the very nature of our societies and cultures cannot be entirely foreseen or predicted. However, discussion of the possibilities with the regard for basic values toward respect for the individual and of dignity of human life will aid us in developing a society that is responsive to the needs of all its members.

CHAPTER SUMMARY

As a result of the increasing use of computers and computer systems, computer crime has become a national concern. Legislation has been enacted on both federal and state levels to protect organizations from unauthorized access to information and computer systems. At the present time, however, it is often difficult to detect computer crime.

Increasing awareness of the existence of the problem will help alleviate it. The types of computer crime that have been uncovered are discussed in this chapter along with discussion of the impact of computer crime on medical environments.

Policy guidelines, implemented and followed consistently, can be instrumental in deterring the occurrence of computer crime within an organization. Proper training of employees is required in order to continue to protect the individual's right to privacy and maintain the special relationship between health care providers and their patients.

TERMINOLOGY AND REVIEW EXERCISES

Essential Vocabulary

computer crime
software piracy
bootleg software
site license
computer hackers
embezzlement
time bombs
data diddling
salami shaving
scavenging
trap doors
trojan horses
computer viruses
computer data theft
computer time theft
wiretapping
passwords
inventory audits
access
Freedom of Information Act of 1970
Privacy Act of 1974
Education Privacy Act of 1974
Electronic Communications Privacy Act of 1986
biometric security devices
dehumanization
depersonalization

True/False

1. Data security for computerized records is rigorously provided in most health care facilities.
2. Data diddling refers to the manipulation of data by authorized personnel.
3. Most health care professionals recognize the threat of computer crime within their organizations.
4. Computer crime may involve computer equipment, computer software, or computer generated data.
5. Protection of the individual's medical record is provided for under the mandates of several federal statutes.
6. The Privacy Act of 1974 restricts access of third party access to information in data banks concerning individuals.
7. The American Medical Association has provided guidelines for the protection of individual medical records and medical data.
8. The use of biometric security devices aids in protecting access to computer data banks.

Fill in the Blanks

1. ______________________ ______________________ involves the infringement of copyright laws.
2. ______________________ ______________________ are individuals who make unauthorized entry into computer systems and their data banks.

3. A ______________ ____________________ must be purchased from a computer software manufacturer in order to allow for multiple use of the software within an organization.
4. ____________________________ is a frequent computer crime, involving the theft of funds from organizations or businesses.
5. ______________________ ______________________ are computer programs that have been introduced into the computer system in order to achieve an unauthorized purpose, whether destructive or not.
6. Satellite communications can be accessed through ____________________ and this is one method through which unauthorized access into data banks occurs.
7. ______________________ are one method of protecting access to information by allowing for only those people with the proper clearance to access data files.
8. __________________________ ____________________ are one method of protecting organizations against computer crime involving equipment theft and loss.

Review Questions

1. Discuss the various types of computer crime that might occur within a health care facility.
2. Discuss methods of providing protection through proper access to computerized information.
3. Identify four laws which protect individual privacy.
4. Define and discuss aspects of software piracy.

Chapter 14

Current Status and Future Directions

Chapter Outline

OBJECTIVES

1. Introduce terminology related to supercomputer technology.
2. Define multiprocessing.
3. Introduce two currently used methods of multiprocessing.
4. Discuss basic concepts in genetic research.
5. Introduce the topic of bioethics in relation to genetic research and computer technology.

The spirit of the pioneers striving to find what lay beyond the next horizon still lives in those of us involved in the computer revolution. We are experiencing a time in history that will see cultural and social changes which reflect the increasing ability of the computer to add to and enhance our daily lives. Estimates suggest that computing powers and speed will increase tenfold in the next few years. Applications will also increase.

New microprocessors are being introduced and utilized to produce faster and more powerful machines. Motorola, Inc. has just introduced a microprocessor chip, the 68040, that will be used in microcomputers and other products. Apple, Inc., Hewlett-Packard, Inc., NCR, and other major corporations will develop product lines using the new microprocessor chips. The 68040 performs at an amazing 20 million instructions per second.

With the first microcomputers random access memory sizes of 64 kilobytes were acceptable and appreciated. Now primary memory sizes of 1 to 4 megabytes are not unusual. The computer industry is producing microcomputers and desktop systems that have tremendous computing power. The variety of microcomputers exist in a price range that make them reasonably accessible to anyone who wants to purchase them. It is not unlikely that in the years to come computers will play as vital a role in our society as the telephone or television.

In our hospitals, computers will come to be considered as necessary as a stethoscope or a blood pressure cuff. Our doctors, nurses, and administrators will wonder how they ever managed without them. The future holds promise of breakthroughs in memory capacity, cost, speed, and increasingly helpful applications that will support patient care.

SUPERCOMPUTING AND MULTIPROCESSING

Up to the present computers have been thought of as reliable number crunchers and report generators. A new stage of development has begun in which the computer is seen as more than a speedy data manipulator but more as an "information refinery." The concept of the computer as an information refinery will expand with the advent of the supercomputing era.

Supercomputers are currently in operation in organizations where massive amounts of computational power are required. These computers generally operate faster than mainframes because of compact circuitry. The circuitry can cover the equivalent of over 50 miles and can process over 1 billion instructions per second. Research institutions, scientific and engineering groups, and other organizations that have complex information processing requirements utilize supercomputing.

Research into the development of even faster and more productive computing machines is well under way. The computer technology being developed today may match or even surpass human intelligence. The technology capable of accomplishing these advances involves multiprocessing.

Multiprocessing refers to linking two or more computers together in order to perform processing tasks at the same time. Multiple central processing units are working together towards task completion through multiprocessing systems. These multiprocessing systems operate simultaneously. Two types of multiprocessing currently in development are coprocessing and parallel processing. IBM Research is working on a parallel processor that will perform 11 billion operations per second. Software designed to utilize the increased computing power of the parallel processors are also in initial stages of development.

Parallel processing uses more than one processor to accomplish a given task. Basically, parallel processing utilizes more than one CPU. Operating systems will be developed to function with the parallel processors to coordinate the activities of the multiple processing units. The parallel processors promise to supercede the power of the first supercomputers which are now in operation.

Coprocessing generally refers to the use of one central processing unit with other smaller, specialized processors working with it. The smaller processors act as "slaves" to the main CPU. The slave processors can work independently and concurrently, performing mathematical computations or other data processing tasks. The main CPU integrates the data coming in from the smaller slave processors.

Multiprocessing systems are not the same as multiprogramming. **Multiprogramming** processing occurs concurrently, not simultaneously. Multiprocessing systems require the use of multiple central processing units. Because multiprocessing involves more than one CPU, they are generally considered to be **fault tolerant**. When components of the multiprocessing system fail there are other backup components available to maintain continuous operations.

Fundamentally, multiprocessing depends upon the very simple concept of integrating and coordinating multiple workers in order to complete the processing task. Assigning more than one worker to just about any task will speed up the process of task completion. Two carpenters can frame a house faster than one, and three can complete the framing job faster than just two. This concept also applies to processing units. If more than one processing unit can be put to work in a computer system, then the processing task will be completed that much faster.

Because the computing power of supercomputer hardware is so powerful, primary storage memory is increased. While personal computers can operate with memory sizes measured in kilobytes and megabytes, supercomputers have primary memories that are much larger. **Gigabytes** measures the amount of primary or main memory in the supercomputers. A gigabyte has the storage capacity of approximately one billion bytes.

The speed of operation of the supercomputers is now being measured in FLOPS, which stands for floating-point operations per second. A **gigaFLOP** capacity refers to billions of operations per second. Soon operations will be measured in **teraFLOPS**, or trillions of operations per second.

APPLICATIONS IN MEDICINE

Genetic disorders can be killers responsible for the development of such chronic diseases as cystic fibrosis and polycystic kidney disease. Victims of cystic fibrosis rarely survive past their 20s. Polycystic kidney disease leads to kidney failure for its victims.

Defective genes are responsible for approximately 4000 genetic disorders. Perhaps as many as one in every hundred born are afflicted with physical or mental abnormalities directly linked to inherited disorders.

Genetic Research and Genetic Engineering

Researchers within the genetic field of study are in the process of isolating the gene or genes that cause many disorders, including cystic fibrosis and polycystic kidney disease. Genetic researchers are also attempting to locate the genetic structures they think are responsible or contributory for such diseases as sickle cell anemia, alcoholism, hemophilia, premature coronary atherosclerosis, retinoblastoma, and colon cancer.

While these endeavors offer hope for the many individuals afflicted with these diseases, they also bring to the forefront many unresolved issues. These issues are the subject of hot debates among scientists and lay individuals alike.

Gene maps are being established by scientists that reflect the DNA structures which hold the instructions necessary for the development of life itself. Sustained by new experimental technology, the inquiry into the genetic makeup of the human body has begun to produce provocative results. Indeed, the National Institute of Health plans research expenditures of billions over the next decade in an effort to analyze human DNA.

Genetic therapy has been introduced in this decade. Gene therapy may act to introduce "healthy" genetic material into the "unhealthy" cellular structure. Hopes for gene therapy include the treatment of ADA deficiency, sickle cell anemia, cystic fibrosis, and perhaps even heart disease and Alzheimer's. Gene therapy can be categorized as one type of **genetic engineering**, the direct manipulation of the genetic structure of a cell.

Genetic testing and counseling is available now in many cases for those patients who have a history of inherited diseases in their family. Testing for the presence of genes can allow doctors to predict the risk of the occurence of an inherited disease.

Tests for disabling diseases such as Huntington's chorea have been developed. Huntington's chorea is a degenerative disease, characterized by memory loss and loss of muscular control; this disease is ultimately fatal. The benefits of identifying and isolating these types of diseases are obvious. The suffering of families affected by these diseases is overwhelming. The desire to have some positive impact on the prevention of these crippling and devastating diseases motivates genetic researchers to move ahead with genetic therapy studies.

The Information Age has arrived as has the **Genetic Age**. In fact there is a complex relationship of interdependency between the two. While Gregor Mendel discovered the existence of hereditary components in the 15th century, and Watson and Crick discovered the double helix in 1953, the trememdous explosion of information relating to genetics has only become possible through the use of computer technology and other sophisticated technological advances. This marriage of the production of medical knowledge and the use of computers in adding to that production is well established.

The advances represent tremendous strides in fundamental principles underlying the functioning of DNA. The study of the action of DNA in the production of proteins which are used as the basic building blocks of the cell could not have been probed successfully without the introduction of high technology research systems that are dependent upon developments within the computer and other related industries.

Preventive medicine may change radically in the future. Disorders may be "targeted" and treatments begun even before symptoms show up in individual patients. Treatments may involve gene replacement or gene manipulation and regulation.

Gene replacement or **gene implantation** will involve implanting genetic material with "corrected" versions of the defective or missing gene or genes. Many disorders are due to a single gene error but others might require identification and correction of multiple genes. Gene replacement can occur in a **targeted cell**, which can be either a somatic cell or a germ cell. **Somatic target cells** are cells that are not involved in the transfer of genetic material from one generation to another. **Germ target cells** are cells that would transfer any new genetic material to future generations. For the present most genetic research involves the use of somatic target cells for gene replacement.

Bioethics and Computer Technology in Gene Research

The term **bioethics** reflects the study and application of ethical systems to biological knowledge and medical technology. As such, the actual field of bioethics can encompass questions concerning the right to life, the right to health care, the protection of the individual, the individual's right to privacy, and even the right to abstain from the use of medical technology that may be perceived by an individual to interfere dramatically with the right to a life with dignity and quality.

Many dramatic questions that have been examined in the field of bioethics have ultimately been resolved in lengthy court battles. Examples of these cases are endless. The family of Karen Ann Quinlan fought a prolonged battle with the courts in order to remove her from life support systems after she had been declared brain dead. Her family believed Karen had the right to die and to die with a certain dignity, that was not to be provided to her by maintaining her body in a chronic vegetative state. The court debate lasted for years while the bioethical and legal implications were considered and studied. Finally, some time after removal of her ventilator system Karen Ann Quinlan died in 1985, almost ten years after the accident which precipitated her hospitalization.

The frequency and complexity of bioethical questions is increasing in the light of the advancements of medical practice. Medicine's ability to preserve life through support systems is increasing. Other medical applications of advanced computer technology, including the study of genetics are bringing many bioethical questions to the forefront. The questions themselves are becoming more and more complex, even asking for definitions of life itself. Further, definitions and explicit guidelines are being sought by health care providers in terms of what their legal, ethical, and financial obligations are in the prolongation of any particular patient's life or in the treatment of any particular patient's disorder.

Financial considerations are increasingly at issue in bioethical dilemmas. Because of the existence of advanced medical technology, the questions regarding allocation of medical resources are becoming more pronounced. Who has the right to receive health care services? Who has the right to receive life-saving, but expensive medical procedures? While our prevailing cultural system suggests that some level of adequate medical care needs to be provided for all individuals, the exact mechanisms for accomplishing this objective have not been satisfactorily implemented. Again, these questions have both legal and ethical implications that may never be totally reconciled.

Bioethics is a field worthy of years of study and individual reflection. The issues are highly complex and interwoven into the very structure of human and cultural values. The purpose here is to introduce the topic with the intent to provide the reader with a glimpse of its relevance in the light of the advances of computer technology.

Computers and Bioethics

One area of study that exemplifies the many questions applicable to the study of computers and bioethics in conjunction with societal impact is that of genetics.

Because the technology is developing that will allow for the genetic manipulation of human cells, bioethical questions concerning the use of genetic therapies are being renewed in an arena that commands both awe and fear.

The term **eugenics** refers to the science of breeding for the development of hereditary qualities. The practice of eugenics in relation to plant and animal life is accepted and employed. In fact, even **genetic cloning** for the development of animals possessing desirable qualities is becoming accepted breeding practice. A genetic clone produces an exact replication of genetic material.

Eugenic practices have been practiced in human populations in the past. Mental and severely retarded patients at one time were sterilized in order to prevent reproduction of "defective" individuals. Historically, more aggressive eugenic practices were found in Hitler's persecution of the Jewish population. These examples raise issues concerning the ability of the human species to use technology wisely and humanely without detriment to its individual members and its own species' genetic diversity.

While the prior examples are clearly reprehensible to most of us, perhaps eugenic practices on a smaller scale are acceptable. For example, reproductive technology today could assist in producing a child of a particular desired sex. Is it not conceivable then that sometime in the future we may be able to control other characteristics of our human offspring? And if so, what effect will that type of genetic manipulation have on future generations of the human species?

For many years geneticists and molecular biologists were dependent upon the expensive computer resources of the mainframe. The cost of the computer's time had to be monitored carefully in estimating research study costs. Now, with the proliferation of microcomputers and minicomputers at such reduced prices and increased power, it is possible for researchers to conduct computer studies with relative ease and at reasonable costs. Without the role played by the computer as a researchers' tool, the advances in research that are commonplace within the genetic field would not be seen for many years to come.

Computer analysis is being used to study the production of viruses that have been genetically engineered. **Genetic engineering** is being employed in the production of viruses for the possible control of AIDS and other infectious diseases. What are the rewards of the successful operation of these viruses? Who can argue the benefit for mankind as AIDS continues to cross international boundaries? Predictions for the number of HIV serologically positive individuals by the year 2000 suggest that many millions will be affected by this disease.

Protein modeling allows for the comparison of protein structures of cells. It is accomplished through the use of computer software designed to help the molecular scientists understand the basic functions of the proteins within the cell itself and is essential to research in genetic engineering.

The promise of genetic study resulting in diagnosis, treatment, and possible cure for disorders is great. However the implications for social problems are somewhat frightening. One of the possible scenarios that is not outside of the realm of belief is that of discrimination based on genetic data.

Any potential carrier of a disease that is prohibitively expensive to treat is at risk for being discriminated against by insurance carriers and by employers. Insurance carriers are already denying HIV positive individuals insurance coverage. Job discrimination on the basis of the presence of the HIV antibodies is commonplace. What will happen when genetic tests exist that can predict the development of alcoholism? or cancer? If corresponding treatments are not available, the individuals who carry the genetic predispositions for these illnesses could conceivably become victims of discrimination in the workplace.

Basically, the reason for discriminatory practices by either employers or insurance carriers is a financial one. Insurance carriers do not want to absorb the cost of treating such chronic, totally disabling disorders. Employers are afraid of possible infection of other employees but they also consider the long term costs in terms of absenteeism or higher insurance premiums when making decisions on whether to retain high risk employees. The legal implications of discrimination against HIV positive individuals is still being tried in individual court cases.

How do these practices apply to people who are carriers of genetically predetermined disorders? Even today with genetic research in its infancy, cases have been reported of discrimination occurring on the basis of the results of genetic tests. It would not be inconceivable for a Health Maintenance Organization or prepaid group practice, for example, to threaten to terminate health care coverage on the basis of information obtained through genetic tests. Undue pressure may be brought to bear to terminate the fetus testing positive for genetic disorders.

Companies involved in genetic testing predict that jobs will be withheld from individuals on the basis of genetic predictions of the onset of disease. As procedures become more and more precise for diagnosis of disorders through genetic material, the potential for abuses against the affected individuals involved increase dramatically.

The responsibilities of health care professionals become particularly burdensome when decisive policies must be set within an organization that has, at times, conflicting organizational goals. The role of the health care provider is to perform services for the patient, which will to some degree impact positively on that patient's health status. While the role of the provider is basically one of service, it is also an action which is taken with the expectation of some financial reimbursement for the actions taken on the patient's benefit.

A conflict occurs for health care providers between the ethical responsibility of providing care and the realistic need for financial reimbursement when individuals are not able to pay for services rendered. Individuals who are unable to qualify for insurance or who for health related reasons become unemployable have no reasonable expectation of being able to pay for health care services.

It seems paradoxical that the very technology that may offer life saving benefits also gives the appearance of threatening the very structure of our health care system. Genetic research and genetic testing will continue. Of that there is no doubt. What we must consider and work towards is developing a health care system that is protective of the individual.

Protection of the right to privacy needs to be preserved in order to maintain the integrity of the doctor-patient relationship and in order to provide health care services to those who require them. Legislation that protects the individual's right to information and protects from access by the vested financial interests of third parties may need to be implemented.

These issues are not to be considered the domain of intellectuals, scientists, researchers, and lawmakers. All individuals must play a part in deciding issues with such tremendous social impact. This fact was recently recognized by the National Institute of Health. Lay individuals must be involved in the effective decision-making that determines long-term research strategies, hospital and other service organizations' policies, and even the laws that govern providers of care. Only with the input of individuals from all levels of our society can strategies and policies which reflect our complex cultural values be established.

CHAPTER SUMMARY

Supercomputer technology is now operational in the United States. Processing powers and speeds are increasing. New computer systems are applying multiprocessing, including techniques utilizing coprocessing and parallel processing.

One area in the health care field that has applied supercomputer technology in research is that of genetics. Computers are responsible, in large part, for the tremendous advances that have been seen in genetic research in the last decade. Computers assist research in identifying genes that are responsible for genetic disorders.

Bioethics is a field of study that applies ethical considerations to fields of biological and medical knowledge. Many questions that are relevant to the delivery of health care are studied through the application of bioethics. Bioethical questions have arisen concerning the use of genetic manipulation and is therefore one area where computer technology is demonstrating a tremendous impact on health care delivery systems.

TERMINOLOGY AND REVIEW EXERCISES

Essential Vocabulary

multiprocessing
parallel processing
coprocessing
multiprogramming
fault tolerant
gigabytes
gigaFLOP
teraFLOP
gene maps
genetic therapy
genetic engineering
genetic testing
Genetic Age
gene replacement
gene implementation
targeted cell
somatic target cells
germ target cells
bioethics
eugenics
genetic cloning
genetic engineering
protein modeling

True/False

1. Multiprocessing refers to linking of two or more computers together in order to perform processing tasks at the same time.
2. Coprocessing generally refers to the use of one main central processing unit with other smaller, specialized processors working with it.
3. A gigabyte has the storage capacity of approximately one trillion bytes.
4. Multiprogramming processing occurs simultaneously, not concurrently.
5. The term eugenics refers to the science of breeding for the development of hereditary qualities.

Fill in the Blanks

1. When massive amounts of computational power are required, the type of computer used is a ______________________.
2. __________ __________ and ______________ is available now in many cases for those patients who have a history of inherited diseases in their family.
3. Gene therapy can be categorized as one type of ______________ ______________, the direct manipulation of the genetic structure of a cell.
4. For the present, most genetic research involves the use of ______________ ______________ cells for gene replacement.
5. ________ ______________ may act to introduce "healthy" genetic material into the "unhealthy" cellular structure.
6. __________ ______________ or gene implantation will involve implanting genetic material with "corrected" versions of the defective or missing gene or genes.
7. The speed of operations of supercomputers can be measured in ______________, billions of operations per second, or ______________, trillions of operations per second.

Review Questions

1. Discuss gene therapy along with its possible benefits and limitations.
2. Describe the difference between coprocessing and parallel processing.
3. What is the difference between multiprocessing and multiprogramming?

Glossary

Absolute cell address—in a spreadsheet, a formula that will not change regardless of its position within the spreadsheet. Absolutes remain constant within a worksheet.
Access—entry into a computer program or data stored in a secondary storage device.
Accounting Information Systems—specialized software that performs basic accounting and business functions.
Action—the THEN section of a production rule in a rule-based expert system.
Active records—records that are referred to frequently or may be currently in use.
Additions—a file maintenance data entry operation involving the placement of a new record within a database file.
Administrative applications systems—in a health care facility includes general accounting functions, financial management functions, facilities management, materials management, and general office computer systems.
Alphanumeric fields—fields that may contain virtually any character on the computer keyboard including letters, numbers, and special characters, symbols or punctuation such as *,#,@, and ^.
Analog computers—work with continuous data transmission, such as sound waves, or volumes. Analog computers process data about measurements.
Ancillary consultation devices—expert systems that provide a means of consultation for the purpose of diagnosis or therapy.
Antecedent—The IF section of a production rule in a rule-based expert system.
Append—see additions.
Applications software—software that performs a specific data processing function for the end user.
Architecture—describes how the central processing unit and its interrelated elements are structured.
Argument—a designated group of adjacent cells within a spreadsheet.
Arithmetic-logic section—performs processing operations on the entered data. These processing operations can be either arithmetic or logical operations.
Arrhythmia monitoring—a standard type of computerized medical instrumentation used in emergency rooms, operating rooms, and intensive patient care areas, providing basic monitoring or diagnostic support for patients.
Artificial intelligence—an applied science involved in the study and development of technology that possesses a demonstrable ability to imitate the characteristics of human processes such as perception, movement, intuition, communication, and decision-making.
Ascending alphabetic sorts—starting with the first letter of the alphabet and proceeding through until the last letter

in the sequence is covered, such as A,B,C, . . . X,Y,Z.
Ascending numeric sort—starting with the smallest number and proceeding through to the largest numeric value, such as the sequence 1,2,3 . . . 7,8,9,0.
Asynchronous transmission—refers to bytes being moved one at a time.
Attributes—column in a relational data base.
Audit trails—a method used to mark and track claims that have not been paid.
Automated medical instrumentation—equipment that operates through electronic means to provide input via measurements and performs data collection and data analysis tasks.
Automated medical record—computerized medical record.
Automated medical instrumentation systems—computerized systems that allow for the complete maintenance of a patient in some aspect of their care.
Backup file—a copy of the file that is created in order to protect data or programs from possible data loss.
Bandwidth—a measurement that refers to the number of bits that may be carried over a communications line.
Bar code reader—see bar code scanner.
Bar code scanner—an optical recognition device that recognizes bar code product labels.
Batch processing—a type of offline processing frequently used in payroll processing.
Baud—a measure of the speed of communications transmissions; bits per second.
Bedside patient management systems—patient bedside monitors that offer noninvasive, continuous monitoring of patients in critical care areas.
Binary digit or bit—the smallest piece of information that can be processed by a computer. A bit can take one of two forms: 0 or 1.
Bioethics—the study and application of ethical systems to biological knowledge and medical technology.
BIOETHICSLINE—informational database system that contains references pertaining to religious, philosophical, and legal issues.
Biometric security devices—security devices that use electronic technology to guard against unauthorized entry into a protected area or computer system.
Bits per second (bps)—measurement reflecting the speed at which bits are transmitted.
Block operations—an operation that usually involves marking more than one character for the purpose of moving, copying, or searching.
Bootleg software—software that has been obtained through unauthorized copying of a computer program.
Broadband—a bandwidth measurement that transmits at a line speed over 9600 bps used when high speed of transmission is required along with the transfer of large amounts of data.
Byte—equivalent to one character.
Calculate—a data processing operation that performs mathematical calculations.
Cardiorespirography—an automated method to detect alarm parameters in either heart rate or respiratory rates.
Cathode ray tube (CRT)—a television-like screen that displays processed information.
Cell—the intersection of a row and column representing a physical location on a spreadsheet.
Cell address—the unique location of the cell within the worksheet, specified by the exact number and character location.
Cell coordinates—the exact number and character in a worksheet that identifies the location of a particular cell.

Cell entries—or data types, are: labels, values, formulas, and special functions.
Cell location—the exact number and letter associated with the location of a particular cell within a worksheet.
Central processing unit (CPU)—consists of three main sections: the control section, the arithmetic-logic section, and the primary storage section.
Channels—data transmission communication lines.
Character recognition device—an optical recognition device capable of "reading" machine printed or handmade characters.
Character fields—alphanumeric fields that are not used in calculations.
Classify—a data processing operation that groups data in some way in order for it to be meaningful and useful, for example, organizing data into similar categories.
Clinical applications systems—software systems that support patient care.
Clock speed—rate of speed measuring the number of pulses (ONs and OFFs) per second; clock speeds are expressed in megahertz (MHz).
Coaxial cable—broadband transmission method consisting of enclosed wires; type of communications link.
Column formatting—formatting columns within a spreadsheet to meet user specifications, including setting widths for each column, setting right or left justifications, or setting decimal alignments.
Combinatorial explosion—refers to the enormous possibilities and alternatives that must be considered before a decision can be reached.
Command driven software—software that requires the user to use a particular sequence of keys in order to perform a particular operation.
Communication service carriers—public or privately owned communications systems.
Communication pathways—can be very complex within an organization.
Communications software—applications software that is used for the transfer of data from one computer system to another.
Compatibility—term that describes the ability of various components of computer systems to work with one another.
Computer—an electronic device capable of performing calculations and comparisons in a fast and reliable manner.
Computer-assisted diagnosis—diagnosis that has been formed with the assistance of a computer that is preprogrammed to interpret patient data and results in a reliable diagnostic manner.
Computer-assisted instruction (CAI)—computer based instructional system that is concerned with the delivery of basic skills and the acquisition of knowledge. Software applications include drill and practice, tutorial, simulation, and basic problem solving.
Computer-based education (CBE)—education that uses computers as an instructional medium.
Computer crime—illegal acts, including but not limited to theft or embezzlement, that involve computer hardware or software in some manner.
Computer data theft—the use of computer systems to acquire information about an organization.
computer hackers—individuals who make unauthorized entry into computer systems and their data banks.
Computer program—a set or series of instructions that is written by a computer programmer in order to allow the computer to process data.
Computer systems—a group of components, including hardware and software, that work together to complete a particular data processing task.

Computer time theft—the use of computer time for unauthorized purposes.
Computer viruses—computer programs that have been introduced into the computer system that may or may not result in destruction of programs and data.
Computerized medical instrumentation—see automated medical instrumentation.
Computerized clinical monitoring—patient monitoring that may take place with the aid of an automated system.
Computerphobia—symptoms of fear and anxiety experienced when using computers.
Conditional sorts—sort to be performed on a particular set of selected data.
Consult-I—an example of an expert system that employs statistical pattern recognition methodology.
Control panel—roughly equivalent to a status line, giving the computer operator the basic information about the worksheet.
Control unit—that section of the central processing unit that acts as a department head and manages all the operations for the entire computer system.
Coprocessing—computer system that contains large processor along with smaller "slave" processors.
Copy—marking out a block of text and making an exact duplicate of the original data for the purpose of moving it to a new location, resulting in two exact copies of the original text.
COSTAR (Computer Stored Ambulatory Record)—computerized and integrated information system that is undergoing experimental development.
Current Procedures Terminology (CPT)—code used for identifying services such as laboratory tests, examinations, treatments, and operative procedures.
Cursor—a small blinking dash that allows the user to determine the exact location for inputing characters and commands.
Daisy wheel printer—an impact printer that "strikes" the desired characters onto the page in much the same manner as a typewriter.
Data—the raw material; the collection of characters and numbers that are entered into a computer.
Data base—the highest level of organization within the data hierarchy, referring to the collection of information that represents all fields, records, and files; a collection of related information.
Data burnout—see data overload.
Data bus—pathway that transports data.
Data communications—the transfer of data over a particular distance.
Data diddling—refers to the modification of data within a computer system performed with malacious or purposeful intent.
Data entry—an input operation.
Data overload—the possibility that the processing of large amounts of information may result in a reduced ability of the observer to recognize significant pieces of information.
Data processing cycle—the process of input, processing, output, and storage.
Data redundancy—the possibility that output and measurements taken by an automated system may be repetitive.
Data transmission—the actual movement of data across communications lines.
Data verification—a process of proofreading and checking to make sure all changes or additions to a database file are correct.
Database management software—computer applications software that is designed for the manipulation of data within a data base. This type of software allows for creation and editing capabilities, sorting capabilities, and comparing and summarizing activities.

Database software—see database management software.
Decision support systems—software that aids in the decision-making process. In health care applications a decision support system may refer to an expert system that aids in clinical diagnosis.
Dedicated computer systems—computer systems designed for processing information for a single or special purpose.
Default setting—settings that have been chosen by the manufacturer as a standard mode of operation for a particular software package.
Deletions—removing a record from a file within a data base.
Delimiter—a period or a combination of periods that marks the cell address as the beginning of a range.
Demodulation—the reconversion to original digital signals after analog transmission.
Descending alphabetic sort—starting with the last possible letter of the alphabet and returning to the very first letter, such as Z,T,Q,B . . . A.
Descending numeric sort—starting with the largest numeric value and proceeding through to the smallest, such as 15436, 15420, . . . 15000.
Desktop publishing software—generally an integrated software that performs both word processing and graphics functions.
Detail reports—reports that provide listings of every record within a file.
Diagnostic Related Groups (DRG)—a code that groups the patient into a diagnostic category that hospitals use to aid the processing of claims for reimbursement.
Digital computers—computers that process discrete data, using a binary numbering system to represent the data to be processed.
Direct access storage devices—storage devices that allow for retrieval or access of records directly.
Disambiguating—the term AI researchers use to refer to the process of removing or distinguishing between ambiguous factors from a computer program.
Distributed processing—refers to processing which takes place with two or more computers linked with data communication lines.
Distributed processing networks—computer networks involved in distributed processing.
Document file—a collection of related text, figures, and/or graphic displays
Documentation—written material that accompanies purchased software, containing the information necessary for using the software appropriately.
Dot matrix printers—an impact printer that forms characters by impacting small dots onto the paper's surface.
Drug administration systems—automated systems that aid the process of administration of pharmaceuticals to patients.
Drug interactions software—computerized information systems may provide information on medications, their individual side effects and possible interaction effects with food or drugs.
Drug administration systems—automated systems that control the amount of drug administered to a patient.
Edit mode—the mode of operation that makes changes in a cell entry once an entry has been completed and entered into the spreadsheet; allows for making changes in a cell that already holds an entry.
Editing—this functions allows for changes to be made within a document or file. Changes may include inserting or deleting data and copying or moving data.

Education Privacy Act of 1974—legislation that provides the individual with access and the right to challenge any information held by public or private school.
Electronic claims clearinghouses—a service business that transmits a claim to the appropriate insurance carrier electronically where feasible.
Electronic Bulletin Boards Systems (BBS)—computerized bulletin boards.
Electronic Communications Privacy Act of 1986—legislation that protects against the illegal interception of data communications.
Electronic medical record—computerized medical record.
Electronic spreadsheets—software programs that allow for electronic calculations to be performed on designated rows and columns of numerical data.
Electronic mail (E-Mail)—electronic transmission of queries, documents, and messages from one terminal or computer to another.
Electronic claims processing—processing that electronically transfers insurance claims from providers of care to insurance carriers.
embezzlement—a type of crime involving removal of funds from organizations or businesses without authorization.
EMYCIN—auxiliary software tool used in designing expert systems based on the principles used to develop MYCIN.
Encoding software—applications software that allows for the classification of patient diagnoses according to ICD-9-CM standards.
EOF—marks the end of a database file, meaning that there are no more records in that file.
Ergonomics—the scientific study of work and space, including the factors that affect worker productivity and that impact on workers' health.
Eugenics—the practice of genetic manipulation for the purpose of "improving" the genetic structure of a population.
Exception reports—reports that choose or select only those records within a file that show some unique characteristic.
Expert systems—software that acts to evaluate data and make decisions based upon that data.
External compatibility—the ability of different computer systems or components of different systems to work together.
Facsimile—see FAX machine.
False negative—a test situation that reflects the state where a test has given a negative result when the condition being tested for is actually present.
False positive—test situation that reflects a state of affairs where a test has shown a positive result without the condition being tested for actually being present.
FAX machines—automated office systems that electronically transmit documents over communication lines.
Feedback control mechanisms—monitoring systems that provide a method of monitoring the condition of a patient.
Fiberoptics—type of communications link.
Field length—the maximum number of characters available within a field, generally limited by the software manufacturer.
Fields—a basic data category within the data base. Fields can be either numeric, alphanumeric, logical, or memo.
File—the named location of material saved on a secondary storage device

such as a floppy disk; a collection of related records.
File maintenance—a data entry operation equivalent to file updating.
File updating—a data entry operation that involves modifying an existing record by replacing outdated information.
Financial accounting systems—computer systems that facilitate the preparation of accounting information.
Financial analysis software—applications software that can provide a measurement of an organization's viability through advanced analysis of basic financial data.
Financial forecasting—analysis of data that can be used to predict future financial status of an organization.
Fixed disk—see hard disk.
Floppy disks—magnetic disks with a magnetic oxide coating over a thin slice of plastic.
Footers—a page formatting feature that allows for pages to be marked at the bottom of the page for the purpose of identification.
Formatting a document—functions that include methods for setting margins, tabs, line spacing, and other page layout features.
Formulas—mathematical operations directed to occur on entries made in cells of a spreadsheet.
Freedom of Information Act of 1970—legislation that allows individuals access to data that has been stored by the federal government.
Freeware—software in the public domain.
Full duplex transmission—data transmission that can move simultaneously in either direction.
Function keys—keys that are used either in combination or alone to perform various procedures for the end user, such as saving or retrieving a document.
Gene implantation—the process of implanting genetic material into a cell.
Gene maps—maps that reflect DNA structures.
Gene replacement—genetic manipulation in order to change the structure of DNA.
General health assessment systems—computerized patient assessment systems that provide a health screening mechanism.
Genetic cloning—the use of genetic material for the purpose of producing an exact replication of genetic material.
Genetic engineering—the manipulation of the DNA structure of organisms for the purpose of changing their genetic structure.
Genetic testing—testing for the presence or absence of genetic material.
Genetic therapy—therapies involving the introduction of "healthy" genetic material into an "unhealthy" cellular structure.
Germ target cells—target cells that are responsible for passing genetic material from one generation to another.
Gigabytes—a unit of measurement; approximately one billion bytes.
GigaFLOP—measurement used for the speed of operation in supercomputers referring to billions of operations per second.
Global changes—changes which apply to every cell within the worksheet.
Grammar checkers—software that attempts to correct for improper word usage within a document.
Grant management software—software that is available for supporting grant allocation of funds.
Graphics software—applications software used to create pictorial representations.
GUIDON—auxiliary software tool that facilitates the use of MYCIN as a teaching tool.

Half-duplex transmission—Data transmitted in two directions, either to or from a terminal.
Hard copy—printed material.
Hard disk—a sealed, dust free container holding a read/write head, an access arm, and a magnetic disk for storage.
Hard hyphen—a hyphen that retains its position in the word regardless of the position of the word within a line.
Hard page breaks—a software feature that controls page positioning by allowing the end user to determine what information will be produced on any particular page.
Hard returns—a word processing feature that marks the end of a paragraph or inserts a blank line within a document.
Hardware—the actual physical equipment that is used by the computer system to process data.
Headers—a page formatting feature that allows a page to be printed with identifying information appearing at the top of the page.
Health assessment system—automated systems that aid in the determination of a patient's health status or aids the health care provider in determining the patient's need for health care services.
Health care research information systems—software systems used to facilitate the analysis of health care research.
HELP system—experimental integrated computer system is operating at the Latter Day Saints Hospital in Salt Lake City, Utah.
Heuristics—mechanisms for simplifying choices and guiding the direction of a decision making process.
Hierarchical data base—a type of data base in which records are related in a one-to-many fashion.
Holter monitoring—automated ambulatory electrocardiography.
Horizontal communications—directional flow that represents communications occurring from the lower level up to the higher levels.
Hybrid computers—computers that process both continuous and discrete types of data.
Hyphenation—a word processing feature that allows for the proper positioning and control of hyphenation when needed for word division.
I/O devices—computer hardware that functions or operates as either an input or output device.
ICD-9-CM (International Classification of Diseases)—classification system for diseases, recognized as a standard for diagnosis coding.
ILIAD—a commercial computer based educational program designed to teach clinical problem solving skills.
Impact printers—printers that produce printed material by making direct contact with the printing surface.
Inactive records—records that are not currently in use but need to be maintained for reference purposes.
Inference engine—see reasoning engine.
Information—output; the result of data that has been processed in some manner.
Information services—services that allow subscribers access through data communications to large data banks.
Information system—consists of input and output, the computer system components, and the people who use the processed data in various tasks.
Inkjet printers—nonimpact printers that shoot out ink in dots onto the paper, capable of producing high quality color graphics.

Inpatient pharmacy systems—computer systems can monitor drug treatment dosages, drug-food, or drug-drug interactions, and regulate administration of intravenous preparations.
Input—entering data into the computer system.
Input device—hardware which functions to enter data into the computer system.
Insert—an operation that involves adding a record between two existing records.
Insert mode—a mode of operation that allows for text to be "added" to a document by positioning the cursor in the correct location and then keying in the additional material.
Integrated computer systems—computer systems that allow for more than one function to be performed, such as both physiological and respiratory functions. Integrated systems can also refer to computer systems that utilize a common data base. Because of the utilization of a common data base, the storage of information is not repeated in different locations from one department to another within a health care facility.
Integrated software package—applications software that contains capabilities for performing more than one application.
Interactive processing—online processing that provides direct and immediate processing after input.
Interfaced system—computer systems allow for the transfer of data from one system to another. The output from one system may be used as input for the other.
Internal compatibility—the ability of the computer system to work together with all of its parts.
Internist/Caduceus—an expert system developed initially by Harry Pople and others at the University of Pittsburgh.
Inventory audits—method of security for computer systems that provides for inspections at unscheduled intervals in order to protect data and program files.
Inventory control software—software that aids in materials management functions.
Justification—a page formatting feature that allows for alignment of margins.
Key fields—fields that may be utilized by any one sort procedure or a field that aids in identification of a record within a database file.
Kilobytes—a term that designates storage capability. One kilobyte is equivalent to 1024 characters.
Knowledge base—a representation of all relevant information about a particular problem area and the rules by which a computer program will interpret the data represented.
Knowledge representation—a representation of all relevant information about a particular problem area collected and described in an appropriate computer language.
Labels—cell entries upon which no mathematical operations will occur, either alphabetic, numeric, or special characters.
Laboratory management software—software that has been developed to facilitate management or clinical functions of a hospital or commercial laboratory.
Laser printers—high end output products for computer systems, capable of near typeset quality output and offering varying graphics capabilities.
Lateral communications—directional flows that denote communications occurring from side to side at the same level within the organization hierarchy.
Letter quality—a good print quality that is acceptable for professional production of textual material.

Line speed—the speed at which bits are transferred over a communications channel.
Local area networks (LANs)—computers linked together by communications lines.
Logical fields—fields that consist of either one of two possible values such as True or False, Yes or No, or Male or Female.
Macros—a series of keystrokes that have been saved under a separate filename that can be used and inserted into a document or documents repeatedly.
Magnetic tape—inexpensive type of medium used for permanent storage of data.
Mainframes—large computer systems capable of processing massive volumes of data.
Major sort—the primary field within a sort sequence.
Mark reader or scanner—an optical recognition device capable of reading handmade marks on predesigned forms.
Marketing information systems—software that analyzes purchasing decisions by consumers for the purpose of analyzing and predicting what approach to take to sell products.
Materials management software—operations management software designed to aid an organization in the responsibilities involved with materials management.
Math feature—an advanced feature that allows for limited calculations to be performed within a word processing package.
Mbps—million bits per second.
Medical informatics—the utilization of computer systems technology in relation to medical care and its delivery.
MEDLARS (Medical Literature Analysis and Retrieval Systems) literature database—informational database that allows researchers to conduct literature review on any of their 20 on-line bibliographies.
MEDLINE (Medical Literature Analysis and Retrieval System On Line)—information system that contains over 6 million references on journal articles relevant to health care professionals.
Megabytes—a storage measurement; one megabyte is equivalent to 1,048,576 characters.
Memo fields—fields that can be used to add data that may be unique to a particular record.
Menu driven—software that gives the end user a selection or choice of operations to choose from on screen.
Merge operations—a word processing operation designed to produce form letters.
Microcomputer—a personal or desktop computer.
Microwaves—broadband transmission utilizing high frequency radiowaves; type of communications link.
Minicomputers—one of the four categories of computers based on size: larger than a microcomputer and smaller than a mainframe.
Minor sort—a sort following the primary sort in a multiple sort operation.
Mode indicator—indicates the current mode of operation in a spreadsheet.
Modems—hardware devices which convert digital signals to analog signals for transfer over communication lines or links.
Modulation—conversion of a digital signal to analog.
Modules—subsets of software that perform related functions such as billing and accounts receivable in an accounting software package.
Monitoring systems—automated systems that track physiological processes, graphing or charting data to

provide necessary documentation of the physical process under observation.
Move—marking out a block of text and actually relocating it in another position; a "cut and paste" operation.
Multicolumn output—a word processing feature that allows for more than one column to be shown on the screen.
Multiple sort—the use of more than one field in a sort operation.
Multiplexor—hardware that serves to concentrate messages from several small data communications lines for more efficient transfer through a transmission channel.
Multiprocessing—refers to linking two or more computers together in order to perform processing tasks at the same time.
Multiprogramming—refers to the ability of a computer system to run two or more programs concurrently on the same computer.
MYCIN—an expert system aiding in the diagnosis of bacterial infections and utilizing production rules that was developed at Stanford University in the 1970s.
Narrowband—a bandwidth measurement that transmits at relatively slow speeds, 45 to 300 bps, used typically in telegraph transmissions.
Neonatal monitoring—monitoring of neonates continuously using an automated monitoring system.
Networks—a complex data base structure that is used with larger computer systems.
No fault tolerance—refers to the reliability factor of the central processing unit.
Nonimpact printers—printers that do not make direct contact with the printing surface.
Numeric fields—fields that consist of a number or numbers (0,1,2, . . . 9) that can be used in mathematical calculations.
Numeric formats—a variety of descriptive formats for numeric values, including dollar amounts, decimal amounts, and expression.
Numeric keypad—a configuration of numbers much like that on a calculator.
Obstetrical monitoring—monitoring for obstetrical patients with the use of automated systems.
Offline systems—computer systems that do not provide direct communication with the processing unit.
On-screen formatting—a software feature that allows for the changes made within a document to be shown on the screen.
ONCOCIN—expert system used for management of cancer patients.
Online processing—processing that occurs through a direct connection between terminals and the computer system.
Open ended architecture—a term describing a computer system that allows for expansion at a later date.
Operating systems—set or collection of specialized programs that perform vital functions for control of the computer system. Operating system programs interface and communicate between the applications programs, end users, and the computer hardware.
Operations management—a branch of investigation that looks at organizations and the way their different departments or different groups of personnel perform activities.
Optical disk storage—a technology that allows for storage of data in a very compact manner.
Optical disk storage systems—permanent storage utilizing optical disk technology

to provide an on-line record to capture data for the record.
Organizational charts—a method of documenting the information flow in an organization.
Orphans—a term describing the situation where a new paragraph begins on the last line of a printed page.
Output—a data processing operation; the final product of the data processing cycle, after data has been processed by the computer system.
Pagination—the ability of a word processing package to allow for control of page numbering.
Parallel port—transfers data by groups or chunks.
Parallel processing—computer system that utilizes multiple processors that are integrated to perform together to complete data processing operations.
Parallel transmission—data communication that occurs when data is transferred by transmitting all bits in a byte at one time.
Passwords—one method of providing security for computer systems that allows only authorized users access to computer programs and data.
Patient bedside monitors—modular physiological monitoring system that tracks the physiological processes of a patient.
Patient computer-assisted instruction—computer instructional system used to facilitate aspects of patient education.
Patient identification variables—variables that identify the patient, including the name of the patient, the patient's social security number, the patient's address and phone number, the patient's employer, and the name of any insurance carriers under which the patient is covered.
Patient insurance variables—variables that include the identification numbers of insurance policies, the categories of insurance that provide coverage for the patient and the structure of any private policy that covers the patient.
Patient maintenance systems—a type of special purpose system that offers complete automation of some aspect of patient care.
Patient scheduling software—software that performs patient scheduling functions for a hospital or clinic.
Peripherals—a category of hardware; the physical equipment used together with the computer for performing data processing tasks.
Physician data query-communication system—example of an expert system.
Physiological monitoring systems—computer systems that monitor physical processes, such as analyzing blood or other fluids. These systems sometimes alert staff when levels reach a need for clinical action.
Pointer—used as a field within an indexed file in order to establish and maintain the sequence of records as they existed in the original file.
Practice management systems—software applications that automate billing and accounting functions for a physician's practice.
Practice specific systems—software applications that apply only to specialty practices such as dental offices, radiology offices, psychiatric practices.
Precedence—term that designates the rules of order for mathematical operations.
Primary memory—the section of the CPU that stores data and program instructions; it does not perform any of the logical operations.

Primary sort key—determines the data by which the first sort on a file will be performed.
Primary storage—see primary memory.
Printing—a function that allows for the page or document to be printed onto paper or other surfaces (such as transparencies).
Privacy Act of 1974—legislation that protects the individual from misuse of data collected.
Problem-solving computer assisted instruction—automated instruction systems that allow the learner to apply problem solving methodologies to a particular situation in order to create appropriate solutions.
Problem specific health assessment software—identifies risk factors for specific types of health problems.
Problem state—in the study of AI a problem state refers to successive and alternative stages in the problem-solving process.
Production rules—one method of knowledge representation where the system is defined by a set of rules based on IF . . . THEN structures.
Production systems—consists of the complete set of production rules that govern a particular application in expert systems.
Prospective payment system—reimbursement systems that allows for the payment of services provided to be determined in advance.
Protein modeling—compares the protein structure of cells with the aid of computer technology.
Provider variables—variables that must also accompany the request for payment of services, including the name of the physician, an identification number for the provider, and information that the provider must report concerning the classification of the patient.
Public domain software—software that is not protected by copyright.
Pulmonary monitoring systems—automated systems used in patient respiratory therapy and in monitoring of intensive care patients. These systems deliver precise measurements of pulmonary flow, gas concentration, and respiratory rates.
Query or Inquiry—a data processing operation that allows for access or retrieval from a storage medium.
Quick medical reference or QMR—an expert system built upon the knowledge base of internist, maintaining disease profiles for 591 internal medicine classifications.
Random access memory or RAM—the volatile or temporary memory section of the CPU; equivalent to primary memory.
Range—a designated group of adjacent cells within a spreadsheet.
Read only memory or ROM—part of primary memory that is installed by the manufacturer of the computer system and contains a set of instructions usually concerned with start up procedures for the CPU.
Ready mode—the mode of operation in a spreadsheet that accepts initial data entry into an empty, specified cell.
Real time—see interactive processing.
Reasoning engine—computer program used in artificial intelligence.
Record—related fields, grouped together and organized in the same order.
Record address—see record number.
Record disposal—the fourth and final stage of the record life cycle.
Record distribution functions—functions involved in the distribution of records for

the purpose of allowing individuals within an organization access to the needed material within the record.
Record input—the first stage of the record life cycle.
Record logging systems—system developed to provide a method for locating or tracking records.
Record maintenance—the third stage within the record life cycle concerned with the storage and retrieval of the record.
Record number—the location of a particular record in a file.
Record production functions—functions involved in the production of records, including decision making, referencing, and documenting.
Record processing—the second stage of the record life cycle and includes distribution and production aspects for the record.
Record structure—particular order of fields within a record that does not change from one record to another.
Record tracking systems—see record logging systems.
Records—any recorded data developed and retained as necessary documentation.
Records management systems—computer systems that provide for the organization and control of records.
Records retention schedule—schedule according to which records are retained.
Relational database software—a popular database software for use on microcomputers, where relationships between individual records exist within the database.
Relative cell address—the formula of the cell will change depending on its position within the worksheet. Most cell addresses need to be relative to reflect changing conditions.
Reliability—a statistical measurement that reflects the ability to replicate the same results under similar conditions over repeated testing of those conditions.
Retrieval—a data processing operation that provides a means of accessing data and programs.
Remote concentrators—see multiplexors.
Revise—a data processing operation that modifies data so that it reflect current conditions.
Right justification—a page formatting feature that aligns the right margins so that each line of text will end at the same line space.
Ring configuration—computer network that has no host computer.
Robotic sensory perception—the capability of a robotic device to evaluate sensory input.
Robotics—the study and development of computer controlled devices that are capable of environmental manipulation, sometimes based on the evaluation of sensory input.
Rule based systems—frequently used in AI applications; computer programs that test for conditions and then takes action on the basis of the results of the test.
Salami shaving—theft that occurs when a computer program removes small amounts of money from an organization's accounts and moves the funds into a private account.
Satellites—type of communications link that uses broadband transmission.
Saving—process of placing moving data or information from primary memory to a permanent storage device.
Scavenging—refers to methods of gaining information for accessing a computer system.
Scrolling—a software feature that allows the computer operator to move

quite quickly from one location in the file to another.
Search—a block operation that "looks through" text to identify a particular word, phrase or name.
Searching—a technique used in artificial intelligence that attempts to examine problem states as a methodology in problem solving.
Secondary sort key—determines the key field by which a minor sort will be performed.
Secondary storage—a means of permanent or long term data storage.
Secondary storage devices—physical equipment that allows for permanent storage of data and programs, also termed external storage or auxiliary storage.
Sensing device—compact, high performance devices adapted to the particular data requirements, marking changes in measurements such as temperature, pressure, or other physiological measurements.
Sensor—see sensing device.
Serial transmission—data communications that occurs when data is transferred one bit at a time in a sequential fashion.
Serial port—a data channel that transfers data one piece at a time, sequentially.
Shareware—software that may be protected by copyright but available for use with little or no fee.
Signal conditioners—see transducers.
Signal processing units—automated signal processors that analyze, evaluate, or interpret the input data they receive.
Simplex transmission—data transmitted in one direction only.
Simulations—valuable computer assisted instructional programs that provide the student with a learning experience that closely resembles what occurs in a real life setting.
Site license—a license granted to purchasers that allows for multiple copies to be made and used at a particular location or within a particular organization.
Soft page breaks—a feature that controls page positioning by determining how many lines will appear on any particular page, usually a default setting determined by the manufacturer.
Soft copy—computer output displayed on a monitor.
Soft hyphen—a hyphen that may not be retained by the software program if its positioning on the line changes.
Soft returns—a word processing feature that marks the end of a line, changing its position automatically if text is later inserted or deleted.
Software—equivalent of a computer program or programs.
Software piracy—the illegal use of software involving the infringement of copyright laws.
Somatic target cells—cell targets for genetic manipulation that is not responsible for passing genetic material from one generation to another.
Sort—a frequently used data processing operation that arranges data in a particular sequence or order.
Source documents—documents that provide the basic data to be entered into the computer system.
Special functions—allow for particular operations, such as averaging, to occur on a single cell or a combination of cells within a spreadsheet.
Special purpose systems—systems that provide services other than strictly medical, nursing, and/or administrative.
Specialized Information Systems—specialized systems, developed to meet unique organizational needs.

Spell check—a software feature that provides a proofreading function for identification of misspelled words within a document file.
Spreadsheet software—computer applications packages that act as "number crunchers" because of their mathematical processing capabilities.
Staff scheduling software—software that performs staff scheduling functions for a hospital or clinic.
Stand-alone software—software packages with only one main application available for use.
Star configuration—computer network consisting of a host or main computer connected to one or more smaller computers.
Statistical pattern recognition—an example of an expert system that defines a problem area, develops lists of possible features that could be present, and relates them in a probablistic manner to possible disease categories.
Status line—mechanism that informs the end user, giving information on page location, line number, and space position of the cursor.
Storage—a data processing operation that stores data and procedural instructions within the CPU.
Summary—a data processing operation that reduces data into a more compact and functional form.
Summary Reports—reports that involve counting and totaling different fields within the file records.
Supercomputers—the fastest, largest, and most expensive of the four classes of computers currently being manufactured.
Synchronous transmission—refers to a group of bytes being moved at one time.
System assessment and analysis—first stage within the system life cycle.
System design—second stage within the system life cycle.
System evaluation and maintenance—final stage within the system life cycle.
System implementation—third stage within the system life cycle.
System life cycle—a number of steps followed in order to design and implement an information system within an organization.
Systems analyst—a professional with specialized computer training that designs and implements computer systems.
Systems software—software concerned with the control and operation of the computer system. It directs, commands, schedules, and oversees the data processing functions to be performed.
Targeted cell—a cell marked for genetic manipulation.
Technostress—the anxiety associated with learning and adapting to a new technology.
Telecommuting—refers to the use of computer systems by workers at home.
Teleconferencing—two way communication between individuals from two or more locations.
Telephone lines—voiceband line consisting of pairs of wires jointed into a cable; type of communications link.
Templates—a software feature available in word processing and in spreadsheets that is used for designing and saving forms that may be reused over and over again.
TeraFLOP—measurement used for the speed of operation in supercomputers referring to trillions of operations per second.

Thesaurus—a software feature used to identify words with similar meanings.
Time bombs—computer programs designed to change or erase data, set up to begin operating at a particular time.
Transducers—convert the basic signals picked up by a sensing device into other more readable forms, possibly calculated and produced through a central processing unit.
Trap doors—entry mechanism into a computer program that may involve unauthorized access.
Tree structure—resembles an organizational chart where the top level record is called the parent record and is related in some manner to each of the lower level records which are called child records.
Trojan horses—concealed programs that allow for unauthorized access into a computer system.
Turing test—an experimental test designed to demonstrate the ability of a computer system to display attributes similar to human intelligence.
Turnkey respiratory function systems—automated systems that provide complete pulmonary function analysis.
Tutorials—a type of computer assisted instruction.
Undelete—a procedure that removes a logically deleted record and returns it to its original place within the file.
Update—a modification of data in order to bring it up to date.
User-friendly—a descriptive term suggesting that a particular software package is easy to learn and use.
Validity—a statistical measurement that reflects a true or accurate state of affairs. Validity measurements may assess the ability of the automated equipment to actually assess a true statement of affairs.
Value added carriers—communications carriers that group data into "packets" for transmission and may be cost effective for large data volumes.
Vertical communications—directional flow that represents communications occurring for the higher levels down to the lower levels in an organization.
Video display terminals (VDTs)—terminals that contain an input keyboard and monitor for viewing output.
Voice mail—electronic mail message system that is capable of processing voice input.
Voice synthesis—electronic output that imitates human speech.
Voiceband—a bandwidth measurement that transmits at a line speed range of 1800 to 9600 bps, used in telephone or voice transmissions.
Widows—a term describing the situation where a line of text that is the end of a paragraph ends on a new page of printed text.
Windows—a feature that allows for more than one file or more than one application to be accessed simultaneously.
Word processing software—a computer application that allows the user to format and edit documents before printing.
Word wrap—the process by which you control the formatting of your document and "decide" where each line should end.
Worksheet—a configuration of empty rows and columns in a spreadsheet.
Zero down-time—a term that refers to a high rate of availability of the central processing unit.

Appendix A: Introduction to Disk Operating Systems

This section is to be used as a short introduction to a limited number of DOS commands. It covers how to:

1 access or load DOS,
2 use basic DOS commands to format disks, call up directory information, copy files, back up files, and delete files,
3 use other DOS commands to create, access, and remove subdirectories when working with a hard disk, and
4 explain frequently encountered error messages.

Complete textbooks are devoted to DOS applications and short courses are available that teach basic and advanced DOS applications. These options should be considered by anyone wanting increased proficiency in DOS operations. It is also useful when learning DOS commands to try the commands out with both a floppy disk system and a hard disk system if both types of computer systems are available for use.

Once the computer system is turned on, the first thing that a computer system must accomplish is loading the disk operating system into random access memory. This process is also referred to as **booting up**. Recall that the operating system is a type of systems software that directs and manages the various operations of the computer system and that the system must have an operating system in order to run applications programs. Most microcomputer systems use MS-DOS as their operating system.

NOTE: For computers that are not IBM or IBM compatibles or that do not use DOS, another set of directions may be required in order to load the operating system.

ACCESSING THE DISK OPERATING SYSTEM

The operations required to load DOS into random access memory (RAM) will vary depending on whether or not the computer system being used has a hard disk drive or is operated with floppy disk drives.

Booting Up with a Hard Disk

When a computer system is turned on that has DOS already installed on a hard disk, the computer system will access or locate the disk operating system on the hard disk and load it automatically. This is one feature that makes hard disks especially convenient. The hard disk storage saves quite a lot of time when accessing and loading programs.

Look for the on/off switches on the computer system. One switch may turn on both your monitor and your computer or there may be two separate switches. The printer will generally be controlled by its own switch. Locate these control switches and turn them on.

Once the computer system is turned on the computer will load DOS from the hard disk into RAM. When this has been accomplished, the computer system will show on the screen a **prompt**, which tells the operator the system is ready to accept a command. Usually the prompt with a hard disk system is the C prompt. The C prompt will appear on the screen as C>__. Occasionally it will be another letter, such as M>__ or D>__. These prompts usually indicate that the microcomputer is linked to a larger computer system. The cursor follows the prompt, as shown. This prompt tells the operator that the computer system is ready and waiting for input.

DATE and TIME Prompts. Usually on a hard disk system the prompt will come up automatically. If using a dual drive system or when the prompt is not the first thing seen on the screen, it may be necessary to enter in some information about the date and time via your keyboard.

The DATE Prompt The computer system will show on the screen: Enter new date (mm-dd-yy):__

At this point key in the new date using numeric keys for the month, day, and year. For example, February 3, 1994 would be keyed in as 02-03-94. Use either hyphens, slashes, or periods to separate the month, day, and year. After the date is entered, let the computer know that this operation is completed by pressing the return or ENTER key—located where the *carriage return* would be located on a typewriter. Note that ENTER and RETURN will be used interchangeably.

The TIME Prompt The computer system will also prompt for the time after the date entry has been completed. It will give the current time according to its internal clock and ask for the new time by showing on the screen: Enter the new time:__

The time on a computer system is based on a twenty-four hour clock. For example, for the time of 6 p.m., add 12 to 6, and type in the number 18:00. Again, after the time is entered, press the ENTER key to let the computer know the operation has been completed.

If working with a single-user microcomputer system and not on a large system that requires logging in, some users prefer to simply press the RETURN or ENTER key without keying in either the date or the time. Frequently however, applications programs will allow access to the current date and insert it into the documents when needed, so many users prefer to key in this data.

Booting up with a Dual Drive System

The operations to load DOS are a little different with a dual drive or floppy disk microcomputer system. The steps to follow in loading DOS into random access memory are:

1. Insert the DOS system disk into drive A.
2. Follow the instructions above regarding the date and time prompt.
3. When the A prompt is displayed on the monitor screen DOS has been loaded into RAM, and the operating system is ready to accept commands.

THE FORMAT COMMAND

Data is stored on floppy 5 1/4" diskettes or 3 1/2" plastic encased diskettes. Before any data can be stored on a disk, however, it must first be formatted. It is possible to buy preformatted diskettes, but most individuals format diskettes for their own use.

Formatting divides the diskette into tracks and sectors so that data can be easily located and accessed when necessary. It is important to remember that the process of formatting a diskette automatically erases everything on the diskette.

New diskettes must be formatted before they can store data. However, previously used diskettes may be formatted also. When reformatting a diskette, make sure that the files on the diskette do not need to be saved.

Formatting Using a Hard Disk System

1. Insert the disk to be formatted into drive A.
2. At the C prompt, key in the words FORMAT A:
   After pressing the ENTER key the computer system will format the diskette and give information concerning the diskette that has been formatted.
   The screen will look something like this:

   Insert new diskette for drive A:
   and strike enter when ready

3. At this point press the ENTER key.
   After the formatting operation is complete, the screen will provide some information about the operation you have completed.
   For example,

   362496 bytes total disk space
   362496 bytes available on disk

   Format another (Y/N)?
4. At the "format another" prompt, enter Y if another diskette is to be formatted. Enter the letter N if no more diskettes are to be formatted.

Formatting Using a Dual Disk Drive System

1. Insert the DOS diskette into Drive A. Turn on the system.
2. Insert the disk to be formatted into drive B.
3. At the A prompt key in the words FORMAT B:
4. After keying in the DOS Command respond to the screen prompts as necessary, then press the ENTER key.

THE DEFAULT DRIVE

The concept of the default drive becomes important in DOS operations. The **initial default drive** is the drive that appears on the screen when DOS is loaded. Therefore, if the computer system boots up to a C or D prompt, then the initial default drive would be either C or D. If the computer system first boots up to the A prompt then the initial default drive for that system is A.

Changing the Default Drive

It is possible to change the default drive. If another drive is to be used as the default simply type the letter of the drive to be used, add a colon, and press enter. For example, if the system is at the C prompt and the default drive needs to be the A drive, type A: and press the enter/return key.

Drive Specifiers

When using DOS commands frequently it is necessary to add what is referred to as a **drive specifier**. A drive specifier allows the user to tell DOS exactly where, on what drive, the command is to be performed. When a drive specifier is not added to a DOS command DOS automatically assumes the command is to be performed on the default drive. The default drive is always the current drive in which the computer system is operating.

Consider the following example. After booting up when using a hard disk computer system the initial default drive of C is automatically determined. At this point typing in the DOS command, DIR, and pressing the return key will result in obtaining a listing of all files currently stored in the C drive, the hard disk.

Still using a hard disk system change the default drive to A, and press RETURN. This procedure changes the default drive to A. The A drive is the current drive so it automatically becomes the default drive. If the DIR command is keyed in at this point the screen will list all files currently being held in storage on the A drive.

To perform a similar operation with a floppy disk system boot up to the default drive, A. At the A prompt type in the DOS command DIR and press ENTER. The screen will show all currently stored files in drive A. To change the current default drive, at the A prompt type in the characters B: and press ENTER. At the B prompt, type in the DOS command DIR and press ENTER. The screen will give a listing of all files currently being held in storage on drive B.

Up to this point DOS has assumed the default drive. However, it is possible to specify the drive to use with the DOS command. To call up the directory of a drive other than the default or current drive, specify the drive to use in conjunction with the DOS command.

For example if the current drive is A, at the A prompt keying in the command DIR B: and pressing enter will give a listing of the currently stored material in drive B.

THE DIRECTORY COMMAND

The directory command allows the user to produce a listing of all file specifications on a storage device. **File specifications** consist of file names and file extensions separated by a period. Use the directory command frequently to identify which files are located on the floppy diskettes.

Besides the file specifications listing the directory command will give other information as well, including the size of the file in bytes and exactly when the file was created. At the end of the directory listing it will tell the number of files that are located on the disk and additionally, the amount of disk space left on the diskette.

Using the Directory Command with a Dual Drive System

After starting the system access the directory listing of the files located on the DOS diskette by completing the following steps:

1. Insert the DOS diskette into drive A.
2. At the A prompt, type in DIR.
3. Press the ENTER key.

Using the Directory Command with a Hard Disk System

After starting the system, complete the following steps:

1. Insert a DOS diskette into drive A.
2. At the C prompt type in A: then press the ENTER key. (This changes the default drive from C to A.)
3. At the A prompt type in DIR
4. Press the ENTER key.

The directory listing of all the files on the DOS diskette will be displayed on the monitor. The listing will continue until all file specifications have been displayed. If more files exist on a diskette than can be displayed on the screen at one time, the screen will **scroll** with the first files being moved off the screen until all files have been displayed.

When looking at the file names displayed on the screen, note the information given by using the directory command. The file name and its extension are listed. Note that the commands on the DOS diskette generally end with extensions such as EXE, COM, or SYS. These extensions are used to indicate program files or the files that operate the software program in use. In most instances these files should NOT be removed from the diskette.

The number that is listed after the file name and its extension refers to the number of bytes that the file contains. The date and time following the size of the file refers to when that file was created or modified.

When the DIR command is used, frequently there are a large number of files on the diskette, more than can be seen on a monitor at any one time. Because of this DOS will continue to add files to the bottom of the screen. The files listed at the top will scroll, or move off the top of the screen.

Variations on the DIR Command

In order to view the file specifications it is necessary to control the movement of the files across the screen. It is possible to do this using a modified form of the DIR command. DIR/P will cause DOS to enter the listing on the screen until the screen is completely full.

When this happens the listing will pause and the bottom of the screen will provide a prompt. The prompt reads:

Strike a key when ready . . . _

This pause option allows the computer operator to view each screen until the required information is located. DOS will continue to show a screen of file specifications until all files have been listed. When the listing has been completed DOS will return to the current drive prompt.

Another variation of the DIR command that is very useful is the wide screen display. The command DIR/W will display all file specifications on the screen without the number of bytes, the date, or the time shown. This wide screen display moves across the screen from left to right, modifying and compressing the available information from the DIR command so that it can be viewed on a single screen.

DOS Parameters for the DIR Command

The /w and /p used in the DIR command are referred to as parameters. A parameter acts to modify a DOS command in a specific way. The use of parameters is optional with DOS commands. They are helpful in that they extend the function of the command.

THE DISKCOPY COMMAND

The DISKCOPY command is used to complete two operations. First, this command allows a diskette to be formatted. (The diskette can be either a new diskette or one that has been previously used. If it has been used, be sure the data on the diskette is of no further use.) Second, this command—in addition to formatting—will copy all files from one diskette to another. The DISKCOPY command will transfer all information to the new diskette, including any information located in hidden files.

The DISKCOPY command requires identifying the **source** diskette and **target** diskette. The source diskette contains the files to be copied. The target diskette is the diskette that is to receive the copied files.

To execute the DISKCOPY command on a dual drive system:

1. Insert the DOS diskette into drive A:
2. Type Diskcopy A: B: at the A prompt.
3. Press Enter.
4. The following information will be on the screen:

   Insert Source diskette into drive A.
   Insert Target diskette into drive B.

5. Follow the directions on the screen by inserting the proper diskettes into the appropriate disk drive.
6. Press ENTER.

On a hard disk drive system with a single disk drive:

1. At the C prompt, type Diskcopy A: A:
2. Follow the screen prompt.

 Insert Source diskette in drive A.

3. Press Enter.
4. Follow the screen prompt. Insert Target diskette in drive A.
5. Press Enter.

USING AND UNDERSTANDING DOS DOCUMENTATION

One of the greatest challenges for a new computer user is that of understanding and using software documentation. Documentation may look as difficult to master as a foreign language but it isn't. It does take a few tries and a few mistakes before it begins to make sense. Still, it pays off in the long run to spend some time working with documentation and "breaking the mysterious code" with which some documentation seems to be written. The old adage "if at first you don't succeed . . ." is appropriate here.

All DOS commands have a certain **syntax**. Syntax refers to how a command must be written in order for DOS and the computer to understand what it is to do. Different commands in DOS will have their own syntax. The syntax of any particular DOS command is built upon the DOS command itself, the drive specifier to be used, the file specification to be used, and any additional parameters that may be added.

In any description of the syntax of a DOS command certain conventions, acceptable ways of writing the syntax, are employed. If any part of the command syntax is optional it will be enclosed in brackets. One example of this notation might include [/P], referring to the pause parameter that was used in the DIR command. Another example might be [filespec], referring to the fact that the file specification is optional.

The syntax for the DISKCOPY command already presented is DISKCOPY [d: [d:]]. The DOS command is written first. The [d] is in brackets, meaning that it is optional, to be used only when needed. The d stands for the drive specifier. Since the DISKCOPY command syntax allows for two optional drive specifiers, it is in effect telling the user that there are several ways in which to use the DISKCOPY command. Let's apply this syntax to the operation of both a dual disk drive system and a hard disk system to see how this syntax actually performs.

The DISKCOPY Command with a Dual Drive System

Using the DISKCOPY syntax with a dual drive system will give you three options on how to write and use the command. Each will perform in a slightly different way. It is up to the user to decide what needs to be accomplished and to choose the appropriate form of the command syntax.

At the A prompt:

diskcopy	This format tells DOS to perform a diskcopy operation. DOS will prompt the user on the appropriate disks to insert into drive A. Both the source diskette and the target diskette will be used in the A drive. First the source diskette will be copied from the A drive, then the target diskette will be inserted and the copy will be written onto the disk put into drive A. Because the drive specifier has not been used DOS assumes that the drive to be used is the current drive which in this particular instance is drive A.
diskcopy A: B:	Two drive specifiers have been used in this example. Using this form of the command tells the computer that it will make a copy of a disk inserted into drive A and will transfer this copy to the disk inserted in drive B. Screen prompts will tell the user to insert the source and target disks into drive A and B, respectively.
diskcopy B:	In this form of the DOS command only one drive specifier is used, B. When this form of the DISKCOPY command is used DOS will perform the operation at the location of drive B. The source and target prompts will appear on the screen and ask the operator to insert the diskettes into drive B at the appropriate times.

THE COPY COMMAND

The COPY command is an important DOS command. It is a versatile command that allows the user to make copies of file, moving the copy to a new location. The COPY command can make a copy of one individual file, a specified group of files, or all files on a particular disk. Further, it will allow the user to copy files to a particular **device**. A device is a piece of computer hardware that works with the computer system. Examples of devices include disk drives, monitors, and printers.

The syntax of the COPY command is complex, because it allows for so much versatility. The syntax is:

COPY [d:]filename[.ext] [d:]filename[.ext]

Sometimes it is written: Copy source destination.

The most difficult thing to remember about using the COPY command is that DOS must know: 1) where to copy from and then, 2) where to place the files that have been copied. The file specification may include a file extension if the file has one. Otherwise, the file extension is optional. The drive specifiers are optional also but only when DOS knows by default which drives to use.

Take for example the command: A>copy command.com B:. This command states that the file called command.com needs to be copied from the A drive to the B drive. The drive specifier A is not stated here because the file to be copied is found in the current drive. Therefore, it is understood by DOS that is the drive in which to search for the file specification, command.com.

THE DELETE OR ERASE COMMANDS

The DELETE and ERASE commands serve to remove files from the storage medium. The syntax of the DOS command for delete is DEL [d:]file name[.ext]. For an example, suppose this is an existing document file called "thisfile" and it is located on a diskette that has been inserted into drive A.

For a dual drive system with the prompt at A>

1. type DEL thisfile
2. press the ENTER key

The file, thisfile, would no longer be found on the file allocation table of the disk in drive A.

For a hard drive system with the prompt at C>

1. type the command, DEL A:thisfile
2. press enter

Again, the file thisfile would no longer be found on the file allocation table of the disk in drive A.

USING WILDCARDS WITH DOS COMMANDS

The asterisk symbol (*) and the question mark symbol (?) are used by the disk operating system as wildcards. Examples of how these are used will best illustrate the function of the wildcard.

The Asterisk Wildcard

This wildcard, designated by the asterisk symbol (*) allows the operator to direct commands to a group of files, rather than just one at a time. The representation *.* allows for the designated operation to occur on all files located on a particular drive. Files can be copied using the wildcard designated; they can also be deleted; further, directories can be displayed using a wildcard. To specify all files on a particular drive, the *.* representation is used. For example to delete all files on the current drive, the command delete *.* would be used. To specify all files with a particular file extension the filename plus the .* designation is used. To specify all files with a particular filename the designation filename.* is used. Look at the examples that follow in order to examine how the wildcard designation is applied.

The Question Mark Wildcard

While the asterisk is used as a wildcard designation for more than one, or for a group of files, the question mark allows for more specificity. The question mark stands for only one character rather than a complete filename or complete file extension.

It can be used in either the file name or file extension. For example if file names bud89, bud90, and bud91 were being copied from the diskette in the A drive to the diskette in the B drive, the following command could be used: copy A:bud?? B:.

COMMAND	APPLICATION
A:>copy *.* b:	All files on the disk in A drive are to be copied to the disk in drive B.
C:>copy *.txt a:	All files on the C drive with the file extension txt will be copied to the diskette in drive A.
C:>copy budget.* a:	All files located on the C drive with the file name budget will be copied to the A drive.

HARD DISK COMMANDS

To this point, we have discussed how DOS operates computer systems with A, B, and C drives, with the C drive referring to systems that contain a hard disk storage mechanism. When using a hard disk storage device it is necessary to divide the disk into accessible **partitions** that are called **subdirectories**. Subdirectories are created in order to facilitate file management. When the number of files increase to the extent possible using a hard disk storage device it becomes necessary to create and use subdirectories.

There are many ways to organize a hard disk. One simple and commonly used method is presented here in order to introduce the concepts of creating, changing, and removing directories.

Root Directory

Word Processing (wp)	Spreadsheet (ss)	Database (db)
wp.exe	ss.exe	db.exe
first.txt	sec.txt	third.txt

Assume for the example that DOS has been installed in the root directory. In order to install word processing, spreadsheet, and database programs on the hard disk, each in a separate directory, the first step in this operation would be to create three separate directories, one for each program.

To create a subdirectory the **make directory** command is used. At the C prompt:

1. Type md\wp
2. Press ENTER.

The resulting directory wp has been created.

It is now possible to copy program files for the word processing program into the wp directory.

Before any program or document files have been added to the subdirectory it is possible to remove the directory. This operation is completed using the **remove directory** command.

At the C:>

1. type rd\wp
2. Press ENTER.

The subdirectory wp has been removed.

After program and document files have been added to a directory, then these files must be removed before the directory itself can be removed.

After all directories have been set up and program files and document files added to them, it is possible to access directories and to move from the location of one directory to the location of another by using the **change directory** command.

For example if access to the word processing directory is required, then at the C:>

1. Type cd\wp
2. Press ENTER

The prompt will have changed to C:\wp> meaning that the word processing directory has been accessed.

The **backslash** marks the beginning of a **path** which assists DOS in locating program and document files. When reading about the proper format or syntax a DOS command will accept, occasionally the path will be specified as [path]. This specification tells the DOS user that the path should be included in the command being used in order for DOS to locate a file in a subdirectory.

DOS ERROR MESSAGES

DOS users will inevitably run into error messages. Error messages indicate what corrections must be made in order for an operation to be performed. Some of the most frequently encountered error messages will be discussed here.

- **Target diskette may be unusable.** This error message tells the user that there is something wrong with the diskette that has been designated the target diskette. In most cases the reason for the error message is that the diskette contains bad sectors and is defective. The corrective measure to be taken is to insert another diskette in the drive designated as the target.
- **Non-system disk or disk error.** This error message is displayed when the disk being used to load DOS into random access memory does not contain the system files necessary to complete the access operation. The corrective measure required here is to insert a DOS diskette into the appropriate drive.
- **Write protect error.** Write protect error messages reflect that the disk you are trying to write on is protected with a write-protect tab or, in the case of plastic encased diskettes, the write protect notch is in place. Corrective measures here include using a diskette that does not have a write protect tab in place. Usually write-protect tabs or notches are in place for a reason, to protect valuable data or program files from being written over.
- **Not ready error reading drive.** This error message suggests that the drive door latch has not been closed or that the drive does not contain a diskette. To correct, make sure the diskette is inserted properly and the drive latch closed.
- **Bad command or filename.** This message tells the operator that the command has not been entered into the computer system appropriately. This error generally relates to improper syntax usage and may require any number of corrective measures. The command itself may not be entered with the correct

spelling. The parameters may be inaccurate. Check the use of the syntax of the command, the placement of colons, backslashes and slashes, and spellings of file specifications to locate any errors when this message is presented on screen.

Consult the DOS documentation for further explanation or if you encounter other error messages.

Appendix B: Word Processing Exercises

One of the most frequently used applications for computer systems is word processing. This appendix is designed to give an overview of what word processing applications include and how they are performed. Most of the applications presented here pertain to basic word processing functions. These basic functions include creating and saving documents; retrieving, formatting, and editing documents; and printing them.

These basic functions will be available on any word processing software package. Therefore the exercises are presented in a "generic" fashion with no command directions given. Each command structure will vary according to the specific software package being used.

A few advanced features are presented but are by no means exhaustive. These are presented to allow the computer operator to experience word processing features that add to individual productivity and to encourage further investigation of advanced applications.

CREATING AND SAVING A DOCUMENT

Documents are saved by a word processing system using the **file specification** which consists of a *file name* and *file extension.* The file name of a document should reflect something about what the document concerns. Usually file names are limited to eight characters, either alphabetic or numeric. Special characters are generally not used in a file name. File extensions are usually optional and consist of three alphanumeric characters. File names and extensions are separated by the placement of a period (.) between them. No spaces should be left between a file name and its extension. For example, LETTER1.MAR would be a correct format for a file specification; LET 1.MAR would not.

1. Write down the appropriate steps for opening a document file.
2. Write down the appropriate steps for saving a document.
3. Key in the following using a word processing system:

    In order to learn to use a word processor an understanding of basic terminology is helpful. Take, for example, the term WORDWRAP. When you type a letter on a typewriter you must return the carriage in order to start a new line. With a word processor the margins are preset and the word processing software will position the returns in the correct location for you automatically.

The return key on your keyboard is usually marked with an arrow and sometimes is marked with the word ENTER. You use this key when you wish to end a paragraph, insert a blank line, or complete a line before reaching the right margin. Otherwise your word processing WORDWRAP will position your textual material for you. It's automatic and it's easy.

4. Save this document under the file name FIRST.DOC

TAKE A MOMENT

1. What is a file name? An extension? A file specification?
2. How many letters are allowed for file names and file extensions with the word processing software being used?

RETRIEVING AND PRINTING A DOCUMENT

Retrieval of a document means bringing the document into random access memory from a storage medium, usually a floppy diskette. Floppy diskettes are **auxiliary** or **secondary storage devices**. When retrieving a document, while it shows on your display terminal it is possible to add to the document, edit it to make any corrections necessary, or modify it in some other manner.

1. Write down the steps to take in order to retrieve a document.
2. Write down the steps to take in order to print a document.
3. Retrieve the document named FIRST.DOC.
4. Position the cursor at the end of the first paragraph by using your directional arrow keys.
5. Add the following text.

   You have now successfully stored and retrieved your first document. Because you are adding text to the document named FIRST.DOC, you have also begun to learn the process known as editing a document. Editing a document can mean adding to a document; it can also mean correcting errors and changing the locations of text used in a document.

   When you edit or make changes in a document that you have previously saved onto a secondary storage device, it is necessary for you to resave that document so that the document will contain all the new changes you have made.
6. Resave the document FIRST.DOC after keying in the above two paragraphs.

TAKE A MOMENT

1. What is document retrieval?
2. Define document editing.
3. Are editing changes made saved to your storage device automatically? What is the procedure to follow to resave a document?

FORMATTING TEXT

Formatting features allow the end user to modify a document or particular aspects of a document in a number of ways. Basic formatting features include bold print, underlining, changing margins, capitalizing, using the CAPS LOCK key, setting tabs, and centering characters on a page or on a line.

In this exercise three formatting features are employed. These features are bold print, underlining, and using the CAPS LOCK key. These three features usually operate on the basis of a **toggle key**. The toggle key gives the command to start the feature and the same key, pressed a second time, gives the command to stop the feature. This operation is very similar to turning on and turning off a light switch. When the feature is being used it must be turned on. When the feature is not being used it must be turned off. When CAPS LOCK key is turned on, all lowercase letters will be capitalized. It will not capitalize the numeric keys and some other special character keys. Use the shift key in order to print the upper case figures on the numeric keys.

1. Locate the CAPS LOCK key on your keyboard.
2. Write down the commands for using bold print and underlining.
3. Key in the following document using the CAPS LOCK, **bold print**, and underlining features in the appropriate sections of the document. Use single spacing except between paragraphs. Double space between paragraphs.
4. Save the document and name the document TOGGLE.

   TOGGLE KEYS are keys located on the keyboard that allow the end user or operator to turn a particular word processing feature on and off. **To turn the feature on** you press the particular key once. To turn the feature off you press that key again. It's sort of like a light switch; it's either **on** or off.

Formatting: Centering Text

In this exercise the features learned in the last exercise will be used. In addition a new feature, the CENTER feature, will be introduced. Lines of text can be centered across the page, sometimes referred to as vertical centering. The center feature is performed automatically by the word processing package when the appropriate command on the keyboard is entered. The center feature can also be used in conjunction with other features including bold and underline.

1. Write down the procedure to center a line.
2. Center the date on the following document.
3. Center, bold, capitalize, and underline the second and third lines of the document. Remember to turn off bold, underline, and CAPS Lock after completing the entry.
4. Save the document under the name MEETING.

(Center current date)
MEDICAL INFORMATICS MEETING
HEALTH SCIENCES AUDITORIUM ROOM #3

The regular meeting of the Medical Informatics group will be held at the University's Conference Room #3 in the Health Sciences Building on the third Tuesday of each month.

This month's meeting will include a speaker on the topic of "Evaluating Cost Effectiveness of Clinical Information Systems." A question and answer period will follow the presentation.

TAKE A MOMENT

1. CAPS LOCK, bold print, and underline features usually operate by the use of a _______ key.
2. Is it possible to use these features at the same time?
3. When a line of text is centered across the page this is an example of centering _______.

Formatting: Aligning Text at the Right Margin

The Flush right feature allows text to be aligned at the right margin. When this feature is turned on, then the cursor will move to the right margin. As the line is keyed in the text will be entered and aligned at the right margin. When the line has been keyed in press ENTER to complete the command.

1. Prepare the following list using the flush right feature to align the phone numbers on the right margin. On each line key in the name, then the appropriate command for the flush right feature, then finish the line by keying in the phone number.
2. Center and bold the title heading.

Emergency Phone Numbers

Mr. Albert Nelson, Administrator	661-5746
Dr. Henrietta Morgan	742-9932
Dr. Robert Newman	662-9866
Ms. Martha Cunningham, Office Manager	342-5305

Using Default Settings to Format A Document

Default settings are settings that have been used by the manufacturer of the software as standard settings. Default settings are used for top and bottom margins, left and right margins, line spacing (usually single), and tab settings (generally every 5 spaces or .5"). Default settings allow the user to enter text without having to set tabs or margins for each document produced. However, it is possible to change these settings so that a document can be formatted in any number of ways.

Use the default settings to produce the following letter on the word processor. Use single spacing as the format for a basic business letter. Save and print the document.

(Position current date to print on line 15)

Dr. Margaret Waldman
2253 Datapoint Drive
Minneapolis, Minnesota 55545

Dear Dr. Waldman:

After reading your outline on your current project for implementing a computer literacy curriculum for incoming medical students at your university, I felt it would be advantageous for us to discuss your plans for implementation in more detail.

I plan to be in Chicago for the next meeting of the Medical Information Processing convention and I hope that you are also planning to attend.

If so, perhaps we can plan to spend some time together discussing the role that computers can play in providing a well-rounded educational program for students within the Allied Health Professions.

Sincerely,

Ruth Walker, Ph.D.
Department Chairperson
Occupational Health
Madison University

Formatting: Using Page Breaks

Soft page breaks are set by default in a word processing package. Most packages will allow for a certain number of lines of text before inserting the soft page break. If additional lines of text are inserted at a later time the page break will automatically reposition itself until it contains the preset number of lines.

Hard page breaks are entered by the computer operator whenever a page MUST end at a certain point. Imagine, for example, in a multipage document that the writer wants to position a table within the document on a page by itself. Using hard page breaks would allow the operator to accomplish the correct positioning of the table.

Formatting: Working with Textual Material

Formatting features frequently used on a word processing include changing margins, changing tab settings, changing line spacing, and changing justification.

When using a typewriter to produce documents the text on the page is justified at the left margin. All text begins on the same space on each line (unless a tab or indent is used). When this occurs it means the text is left justified. However, using a type writer does not allow for text to be justified at the right margin. The right margin has a jagged edge because each line ends in a unique position depending on the amount of letters and spaces used within that line of text.

Using a word processor allows for right justification. Right justification may be used as a default, meaning that text will be justified on the right of each document automatically. If right justification is by default then it can be turned off, allowing the document to be produced with a jagged right edge.

Again, by default most word processors allow for placement of tabs at each 1/2" or every 5 spaces. Frequently these tab settings need to be changed for the production of documents requiring different settings.

Settings can be introduced at the beginning of a new document and remain in effect until that document is completed. Or in some cases settings will be changed temporarily within a document and stay in effect until new settings are introduced within the document.

Line spacing is also set by default. Most packages use a single line spacing and allow the user to change the line spacing whenever necessary. As with tab settings, line spacing can be changed at the beginning of the document and stay in place throughout the document. It can also be changed within a document temporarily.

Formatting Textual Material Exercise 1

1. Create the following table under the file name ABSENCES.
2. Set Tab settings at 1.5", 3.5", and 6".
3. Triple space between each line
4. Center the heading.
5. Flush right the date.
6. Center the table on the page.

Unit Personnel Absentee Report
Surgical Unit
April, 19____

Professional Category	Number of Days	Percent
Registered Nurses	7	16.6
LVNs	11	26.2
Ward Clerks	14	33.3
Administrative	10	23.8
Total Days	42	99.9

FORMATTING FEATURES FOR RESEARCH PAPERS

Headers and footers mark the pages of a document with information that aids in either the identification of the document or the number of the page within the document. As the names imply, a header places the identifying information at the top of a page. A footer places the information at the bottom of a page.

Footnotes and endnotes are added to research papers or other documents that require additional types of documentation of source materials that have been used in the production of the document.

Formatting Textual Material Exercise 2

1. Set left margin at 1.5 inches. Set right margin at 1.5 inches. Double space.
2. Create identifying header. Add header and pagination.

Robotics in Health Care

Robots have been used for a number of years in manufacturing environments where they have replaced human workers in jobs where the demands are rigorous and the work conditions either tedious or dangerous. It is not surprising that they are currently being introduced as effective health care workers.

Robots are capable of making precise movements, lifting heavy objects, can be programmed to recognize simple voice commands, or even respond to nonverbal cues such as a hand clap. Robot systems are carving a niche for themselves in the health care industry as nursing assistants and even surgical support technicians.

Costs of robotic systems are still exorbitant. A simple robot assistant capable of moving across a room, lifting up to 15 pounds and capable of acting as a personal assistant can be bought today for about $15,000. However as the technology develops, hospitals may find their introduction a cost effective tool for working in such areas as central processing, loading and unloading medical supply deliveries. Other areas where they might be employed could be in delivery of meal trays to patients or even working in areas where hazardous levels of radiation might be located.

The following document will require the placement of footnotes, a header to be placed on page 2, and page numbering on page 2 to be centered at the top of the page. Double space. Save as labor.txt.

Optical Recognition Systems in Laboratory Medicine
by Janine Simpson

Optical recognitions systems have been introduced into the management of clinical laboratories and have proved to be an effective means of processing patient data and test results. Laboratories using these systems have reduced the time required for tests to be run and can run more tests within a specified time period.

Comparisons of the efficiency and effgctiveness of these automated laboratory systems demonstrate without question that even though setting up a laboratory system can be expensive, it is a cost effective technique. Fewer personnel are required to run the tests and, in this way, human resources are optimized.[1]

Automated systems generally utilize the optical recognition device by using a bar code reader to input laboratory specimens into the system. Bar codes are generated for each specimen at the time of request for laboratory analysis that accompanies the specimen to the laboratory. The types of test to be performed are associated with sample identification variables and processed through the automated system.

Some laboratory management systems are capable of evaluating bacterial specimens and then suggesting probable effective treatment regimens that will adequately control the bacteria. These types of systems are exhibiting characteristics of "expert systems" that aid clinicians in making appropriate treatment decisions.[2]

The complete system, including the bar code reader input devices and other computer hardware, together with appropriate laboratory management software function reliably in producing valid test results. Other laboratory functions are being automated as well. Quality control procedures and other administrative tasks have undergone automation. Databases are being generated that maintain and utilize patient data.

1. Brothers, Jerome, "Clinical Laboratory Mangement System." *Computers and Medicine,* Justin Publishing Company, Anaheim, Massachusetts, 1989.
2. Ash, Lauren, *Expert Systems in Clinical Management,* Washburn, Inc., London, 1990.

EDITING TEXT

Editing: Controlling the Cursur

Cursor movement allows the user to move the cursor in order to make corrections, additions, or deletions of text within the document. Generally a number of options for cursor movement are available in each word processing package. The arrow keys located on the right hand side of the keyboard will allow cursor movement one space at a time in any direction.

It is possible to move throughout the document a little faster. Determine the command sequence of the word processing software to relocate the cursor in the following ways.

- to the top of the current page
- to the bottom of the current page
- to the end of a line
- to the left edge of the screen
- to the end of a word
- to the right edge of the screen
- to the end of a document
- to the very beginning of a document

Editing: Modes of Operation

Most word processor operate in an **insert mode**. The insert mode refers to the fact that when letters are keyed into a document the letters will be positioned at the location of the cursor. Any letters that already exist in the document will be preserved by moving them to the right as new letters are added. The insert mode may also be called overstriking. Look at the following example.

The doctors examined the young patient.

Using the insert mode position the cursor at the space between the words The and doctor. Type in the word "clinic." After typing the word in the sentence will read: The clinic doctors examined the young patient.

Now change to the typeover mode and position the cursor at the first letter of the sentence. Type in "A physician." The sentence will now read: A physician examined the young patient. Do not save these exercises.

Editing: Making Corrections

Word processing software allows corrections to be made easily, instead of spending time retyping when errors are made. With a word processor corrections can be made before the document is even printed. Frequently, when keying in new material words can be misspelled. These types of corrections are made quickly and easily using word processing software.

With most word processing packages deletions of letters or spaces can be made with the **delete** key or the **backspace** key. The delete key will remove characters or spaces directly above the cursor location. The backspace key will remove characters or space one space to the left of the cursor.

In order to delete complete words, sentences, paragraphs, or even sections of a page, there are methods to accomplish this using a particular combination of keys.

Determine the command sequences in order to accomplish the following.

- delete a word
- delete to the end of a sentence
- delete to the end of a paragraph
- delete to the end of a page
- delete to the end of a document

Editing: Using Block Operations

Block operations are also considered an editing feature. A block operation allows the word processor to mark off a certain portion of a document whether it is a single word, sentence, paragraph, page, or even a number of pages. When a portion of text has been blocked, then certain operations can be performed with it. For example a block of text could be moved from one position in the text to a completely new position.

The versatility of the block operation depends in part on the word processing package being used, but many packages allow for blocks of text to be edited in a wide variety of ways.

A block can be:

- deleted
- moved
- copied
- changed to bold print
- underlined
- printed
- appended or added to another document

Editing: Using Move and Copy

The COPY and MOVE commands are frequently used in conjunction with a block operation. The COPY command will actually make a copy of a block of text and reposition the copy in a new location. The COPY command leaves the original text in place while replicating the text in a new location. The MOVE command, on the other hand, will perform a cut and paste procedure that actually relocates the original text.

Editing: Search Operations

Search features allow the end user to direct the computer to look through a document for a particular word, phrase, or other defined character sequence. Examples of the use of the search feature include locating a name that needs to be changed within a document, locating a particular word that might have been used inappropriately throughout a document, and locating a sequence of characters such as ###, that might have been used to mark the location to insert text or graphics at a later time.

1. Key in the following paragraph exactly as written. Note that the word monitor is misspelled.
2. Use the search feature to locate each use of the word "moniter." Replace it with the correct spelling, monitor.

COMPUTER MONITERS

Different types of computer moniters can be purchased. A moniter may be available with single color or monochrome screen. Other moniters may show color. Moniters vary in their ability to show graphics.

ADVANCED APPLICATIONS: USING THE SPELLER AND THESAURUS

The speller or spell checker will mark words that are either misspelled or words that are not found within its dictionaries. *Words that are not located in the spelling dictionary of the word processing software that are misspelled will NOT be highlighted.* Using a spell checker is an aid but it is not to be considered a replacement for careful proofreading. Spell checkers are not foolproof; they will not "catch" all spelling errors and will not locate improper grammar usage.

The thesaurus feature will provide a writer assistance in locating words that have similar meanings. Most writers have a tendency to repeat the same word frequently. In order to avoid this tendency a thesaurus is used as a writing aid.

1. Retrieve the exercise named labor.txt and use the spell check feature to check for spelling errors.
2. Next use the thesaurus feature to find a replacement for the word "utilize."

ADVANCED APPLICATIONS: CREATING MACROS

Macros are an advanced word processing feature that allow a computer user to save frequently used keystrokes for the purpose of retrieving and reusing them in the preparation of documents. Macros can involve saving textual material but can also involve saving formatting codes and other commands. Macros are limited only by the imagination of the user.

Creating Macros

Create a Personal Letterhead

1. Turn the macro feature on.
2. Move the cursor to the proper location in order to print the letterhead on line 8 of the page.
3. Center each line of the letterhead.
4. Key in your name, address, city, and phone number following the example below.

Your Name
Address
City, State, Zip Code
(Area Code) Phone number

Create a macro closing.

1. Turn your macro feature on.
2. Create a closing macro that you can use for business letters.

Example:

Sincerely,

(Enter your name)

Inserting Macros into a Business Letter

1. Key in the following business letter using the macros just created. Insert the letterhead first. After completing the letter insert the closing macro.
2. Save the letter under the file name Bonsall. Print a copy.

(Insert Letterhead Macro)

(Insert current date on line 15)

Mr. Harvey Bonsall
Medical Management Associates
515 Circle Drive
Houston, Texas 77006

Dear Mr. Bonsall:

Thank you for your recent letter suggesting that interview with your organization. I appreciate your response to my resume.

At this time I have accepted employment with the Columbus Ohio Health Department as their Data Processing Manager. Therefore, I will be unable to meet with you.

I do hope that you will find a suitable candidate to meet your organizational requirements and again thank you for your consideration.

(Insert closing macro here)

ADVANCED APPLICATIONS: MERGE OPERATIONS

Merge operations involve the production of primary and secondary files so that they can be joined to create a number of standard documents that appear to be individualized. The primary file is generally a letter or document that is prepared with the intention of circulating it to more than one person. With that purpose in mind, individual information is left out of the primary file. The secondary file contains the information pertaining to each individual to which the primary file is to be circulated. The secondary file frequently is a listing of individuals with their names and addresses, although it may contain other pertinent data.

Merge Exercise 1

Primary File. Save this document under the file specification Event.pri.

(Field 1)
(Field 2)
(Field 3)

Dear Dr. (Field 4):

We are in the process of organizing the annual charity event for the benefit of Boston University Hospital. This year we will host a dinner and dance to be held at the fabulous Oak Hills Country Club.

Tickets are available for a deductible contribution of $100.00 per couple. We know we can count on you to participate in this worthwhile event. Please send in the enclosed envelope with your registrations and contribution for the event.

Sincerely,

Anna Gibson,
Event Coordinator
Boston University Hospital

Enclosure

Secondary File. Save this file under the file specification Event.sec.

Record 1:
Dr. Daniel Grayson
3465 Herald Way
Boston, Massachusetts 02109
Grayson

Record 2:
Dr. Marilyn Hodges
735 Byrnes Dr.
Boston, Massachusetts 02109
Hodges

Record 3:
Dr. Marvin Stewart
2499 Bent Bow
Boston, Massachusetts 02109
Stewart

Merge Exercise 2

Another frequent application of merge operations is that of collection requests. Create the following primary and secondary files and then perform the merge operation on the two files. Make sure each field is correctly placed within the primary file. Also be sure that each record within the secondary file contains the same number of fields.

Primary File. Save the following letter under the filename collect.pri.

(Field 1)
(Field 2)
(Field 3)

Dear (Field 4):

It has been over (Field 5) since our office has received a payment on your patient account. We would like to arrange a payment plan with you.

If you can not send the full amount of (Field 6) that is past due, please call our office within the next ten days to arrange a suitable payment schedule.

We understand that sometimes medical bills can be unexpected and want to work with our patients to provide methods of payment that do not involve collection proceedings.

Sincerely,

John Wordsmith,
Patient Accounts Manager

Secondary File. The secondary file will be named collect.sec and contain the following fields: name, address, city and zip code, the name to be used in the salutation, the number of months the account is overdue, and the amount that is owed.

Record 1:
Ms. Adrainne Jones
756 Ivy Lane
Harristown, Pennsylvania 67666-6789
Ms. Jones
3 months
$546.78

Record 2:
Mr. Steven Gonzales
76899 Terrell Road
Harristown, Pennsylvania 67666-6782
Mr. Gonzales
2 months
$245.00

Record 3:
Mrs. Barbara Fredrich
452 Eldon Avenue
Spring Creek, Pennsylvania 67666-6758
Mrs. Peters
4 months
$75.00

Record 4:
Ms. Sally Greer
5678 Spring Meadow
Spring Creek, Pennsylvania 6766-6758
Ms. Greer
3 months
$125.OO

ADVANCED APPLICATIONS: SORTING

Sort operations provide a mechanism through which data can be arranged in a particular order. Sorts can be alphabetical, arranging names or other data in an ascending or descending alphabetical order. Sorts can also arrange information into numerical order. An example of a numerical sort might be that of organizing a list of names and address by zip code.

Key in the following employee listing of a teaching hospital.

Employee List

Name	Specialty	Title
Dr. Edwin Markowitz	OB/GYN	Lecturer
Dr. Marion Stedman	Internal Medicine	Asst. Prof.
Dr. David Watkins	Cardiology	Professor
Dr. George Johns	Endocrinology	Professor
Dr. Julia Edwards	Internal Medicine	Lecturer
Nicole Henderson	Nursing	Asst. Prof.
Mathew Burnett	Internal Medicine	Lecturer
Dr. Bill Bennett	Cardiology	Asst. Prof

Sort the above list in the following ways.

1. Sort alphabetically by last name. (Do not include the title or column headings in the sort procedure.)
2. Sort by specialty all those in cardiology.
3. Sort by specialty and alphabetically all those in internal medicine.
4. Sort by title all professors. Arrange in alphabetical order.

ADVANCED APPLICATIONS: NEWSLETTER COLUMNS

Set for two equal columns.

The Seattle City Hospital is pleased to announce the implementation of several new programs to be offered in conjunction with the Community Health Clinic.

Prenatal care is to be offered at the clinic beginning September 26th. Hours of operation will be Monday through Saturday from 9 a.m. to 8 p.m. The cost of patient visits will be based on a sliding scale fee, based on the patients' ability to pay for services. No one will be turned away because of inability to pay.

The Heart Alert program is to be expanded to include a Smoking Cessation Clinic and a Blood Pressure and Cholesterol Check in addition to the educational program already being offered.

The Smoking Cessation Clinic is open to all interested participants free of charge. Registration will be on a first come basis, as seating is limited. The first clinic will be held on September 31st. Other clinics will be set up for the 1st Monday as well as the 3rd Saturday of every month. The Monday clinic will be held at 7 p.m. at the Community Health Clinic and the Saturday clinic will be held at 11 a.m. at the same location. Register for these clinics by calling 657-9472.

Blood pressure and cholesterol checks will be offered during normal clinic operations.

Appendix C: Spreadsheet and Database Exercises

The first exercise in this section illustrates some basic spreadsheet terminology. Look at the grid below.

	A	B	C	D	E	F	G	H
1	Clinic			Patients				
2	OB/BYN			89				
3	Pediatrics			70				
4	Cardiology			98				
5	Total			(D2+D3+D4)				

Every spreadsheet begins with a grid that identifies rows and columns. This grid is referred to as the **worksheet**. The intersection of the row and column marks the unique **cell location** or **cell coordinate**. Entries into each cell location can be alphanumeric, numeric, or alphabetic. In the above example, locate the numeric entries or *values* in cell locations D2, D3, and D4. Are there any other numeric entries at the present time? Where are the alphabetic entries or *labels*? At what cell coordinates? The entry for the cell location D5 is a *formula,* directing the spreadsheet software to add the numeric entries in cells D2, D3, and D4.

The number of cells within a spreadsheet package will vary according to the particular package used. The more cells available to use in the worksheet, the more calculations that can performed in any one application.

Default settings are used in spreadsheet packages. By default each cell location has an equal number of spaces. The size of the cell, however, can change when necessary to adapt to the needs of the individual spreadsheet.

Loading your Spreadsheet Program

Loading procedures will vary depending on the spreadsheet you are using and the type of computer system being used. The disk operating system must be accessed, however, before the spreadsheet. Your instructor will assist you in loading the operating system and your spreadsheet program. Write down the sequence of commands to follow.

After loading the spreadsheet a blank worksheet will appear on the monitor with the rows and columns marked appropriately. Either across the top of the screen or located at the bottom of the screen, *status line* will be present that gives information about the spreadsheet.

Creating and Saving a Simple Spreadsheet

Creating the Spreadsheet. Complete your first spreadsheet by creating the following worksheet. Mark the cells that are labels appropriately.

	A	B	C	D	E
1	Patient Census				
2	December 2, 19__				
3	Medical Units			Surgical Units	
4	Unit 1	15		Unit 5	14
5	Unit 2	13		Unit 6	17
6	Unit 3	19		Unit 7	13
7	Unit 4	12		Unit 8	20

After entering in the data into your computer system. read the section below.

Saving a Spreadsheet. Spreadsheets can be saved to a floppy disk or to a hard disk by using the appropriate command. A file name and extension must be created for each individual spreadsheet that is saved. It is important to name a spreadsheet file in a manner which will help identify at a later time what information that particular spreadsheet contains. An example of spreadsheet file name might be Jan.bud. Jan is the file name while bud is the file extension. This particular file specification might hold data concerning a January budget for the organization.

Save the spreadsheet patient census as with the filename patient and the file extension, cen. Remember to separate the filename and extension with a period with no spaces in between.

Retrieving and Editing a Spreadsheet

Retrieval. Once a spreadsheet has been saved to a storage media, then in order to work with the spreadsheet again, it must be accessed and returned to the primary memory of the computer system. Retrieve the spreadsheet patient.cen.

Editing Operations In a Spreadsheet. Changes made to a spreadsheet can include adding or deleting columns, adding or modifying existing formulas, and simply correcting any data entry errors.

Make the following changes on the patient.cen spreadsheet.

1. Insert a row between the title of the worksheet and the date.
2. Enter the name St. Mary's Hospital in the new row.
3. Save the spreadsheet with these changes.

Creating Formulas In a Spreadsheet

Retrieve the file patient.cen. Create formulas that will add and total the census figures for the file patient.cen. One total will include the patient census for all medical beds. Another total will include the patient census for surgical beds. The other formulas give an average for both medical and surgical beds.

	A	B	C	D	E
1	Patient Census				
2	St. Mary's Hospital				
3	December 2, 19__				
4	Medical Units			Surgical Units	
5	Unit 1	15		Unit 5	14
6	Unit 2	13		Unit 6	17
7	Unit 3	19		Unit 7	13
8	Unit 4	12		Unit 8	20
9	Totals	(@SUM B5 . . B8)			(@SUM E5 . . E8)
10	Aver	B9/4			E9/4

Once you have entered the appropriate formulas to total and average the figures your spreadsheet will calculate the totals and averages. Note how the formulas were entered in cells B9 and E9. Is there any other way these formulas could have been written? Is there any other way the formulas in B10 and E10 could be written? What are they?

Spreadsheet Exercise 1

Create an inventory/supply spreadsheet using the following format. Mark labels as needed. Align cells appropriately. Format the column for units needed as whole numbers. Save the spreadsheet under the filename supply.

Unit Inventory/Supplies
Hospital Checklist
Date: Unit:
Performed by: ______________

Product Number by Manufacturer	**Supplies Needed**
Invacare	
EJ6374	24
VA7269	5
Health Care Systems	
67-4239	0
43-8872	0
American Hospital Supply	
42364	47
97688	10

Retrieve the spreadsheet supply, add a row under the Invacare Manufacturer, include the new product number EJ5523, and the units needed 15. Print and save the spreadsheet.

Spreadsheet Exercise 2

Creat a spreadsheet template that can be used as a purchase order form. The quantity and unit price will be multiplied to give the amount. Copy the formula entered so that ten lines are available for the purchase order. Insert formula for total amount of purchase order.

St. Louis Health Clinic
Purchase Order
Date:

Description	Quantity	Unit Price	Amount
			Total:

DATABASE EXERCISES

Creating a Database File

Load the database software program. Create the following database file with the following five fields: last name, identification number, primary diagnosis, physician, and account balance. Six records with identifying patient information will be entered initially into the file. Save the file under the name patient.

LASTNAME	ID NO.	PRIM. DIAG.	PHYSICIAN	ACCT. BAL.
Smithson	435672	Hypertension	Waitz	67.00
Johnson	243253	Diabetes	Mitchell	145.00
Weaver	384565	Otitis Media	Mitchell	00.00
Braumum	244879	Hypertension	Waitz	100.00
Zacharey	794543	Cystic Fibrosis	Wright	475.00
Martinez	367546	Obesity	Waitz	25.00

Retrieve the patient database file and print a copy of the original file.

Sorting the Database File

Retrieve the patient database file and sort the data by descending numerical sort on the field containing the account balance. Print a copy of the sorted file.

LASTNAME	ID NO.	PRIM. DIAG.	PHYSICIAN	ACCT. BAL.
Zacharey	794543	Cystic Fibrosis	Wright	475.00
Johnson	243253	Diabetes	Mitchell	145.00
Braumum	244879	Hypertension	Waitz	100.00
Smithson	435672	Hypertension	Waitz	67.00
Martinez	367546	Obesity	Waitz	25.00
Weaver	384565	Otitis Media	Mitchell	00.00

Retrieve the patient database file. sort the data by ascending alphabetical sort, and print a copy of the sorted file.

LASTNAME	ID NO.	PRIM. DIAG.	PHYSICIAN	ACCT. BAL.
Braumum	244879	Hypertension	Waitz	100.00
Johnson	243253	Diabetes	Mitchell	145.00
Martinez	367546	Obesity	Waitz	25.00
Smithson	435672	Hypertension	Waitz	67.00
Weaver	384565	Otitis Media	Mitchell	00.00
Zacharey	794543	Cystic Fibrosis	Wright	475.00

Retrieve the patient database file and sort the data by alphabetic ascending sort in the field containing the primary diagnosis. Print a copy.

LASTNAME	ID NO.	PRIM. DIAG.	PHYSICIAN	ACCT. BAL.
Zacharey	794543	Cystic Fibrosis	Wright	475.00
Johnson	243253	Diabetes	Mitchell	145.00
Smithson	435672	Hypertension	Waitz	67.00
Braumum	244879	Hypertension	Waitz	100.00
Martinez	367546	Obesity	Waitz	25.00
Weaver	384565	Otitis Media	Mitchell	00.00

Retrieve the patient database file and sort the data by alphabetic ascending sort in the field containing the physicians name. Print a copy.

LASTNAME	ID NO.	PRIN. DIAG.	PHYSICIAN	ACCT. BAL.
Weaver	384565	Otitis Media	Mitchell	00.00
Johnson	243253	Diabetes	Mitchell	145.00
Martinez	367546	Obesity	Waitz	25.00
Braumum	244879	Hypertension	Waitz	100.00
Smithson	435672	Hypertension	Waitz	67.00
Zacharey	794543	Cystic Fibrosis	Wright	475.00

Modifications, Additions and Deletions in a Database File

Access the patient database file and make the following changes to the file.

1. The patient ID number for Braumum has been entered incorrectly. Change it to 245879.
2. Dr. Wright is no longer practicing in the clinic. Delete the Zacharey patient record.
3. A new patient has been seen by Dr. Mitchell. Enter the data concerning his new patient: Comfeld, 845365, Strep Throat, Mitchell, 25.00.
4. Save the modified patient database file.

Summarizing Database Fields

1. Use the modified patient database file. Create and print a report that gives all patient data on Dr. Mitchell's patients.
2. Using the modified patient database file, create and print a report that gives the total account balance on all patients.

Appendix D: Programming Languages

Presented here are a number of programming languages that are in use today. These programming lanuages are all considered high level languages, because they are English oriented and operate on a variety of computer systems. Many languages have been developed in response to a wide variety of data processing needs and this discussion is limited to just a few of the major ones.

ADA is a programming language developed by the Department of Defense. One of its primary advantages is that it is designed to run on different size microprocessors. It is also a highly structured language appropriate for use in scientific, engineering, and business applications.

The computer programming language **BASIC** (**B**eginner **A**ll **P**urpose **S**ymbolic **I**nstruction **C**ode), was developed at Dartmouth College in the 1960s and has become the major language used on microcomputers. It was the first interactive program, providing for responses to the user in diagnosing errors in program coding. There are many versions of BASIC. Updates, or newer versions of the language have made it more powerful. BASIC will probably continue to be widely used for years to come.

A machine independent programming language, **COBOL** (**CO**mmon **B**usiness **O**riented **L**anguage), was developed in the late 1950s in an attempt to provide a national standard for programming business applications. One advantage of the language is its easy to understand English-like program statements.

FORTRAN (FORmula TRANslator) has primarily scientific and mathematic applications. It was the first high level language developed in 1954. The language is still in use and popular because of its simplicity for use in engineering.

PASCAL, developed in the 1970s by a Swiss professor, Nicklaus Worth, is widely used for education purposes. It is available for use on microcomputers and is also known for its simplicity.

RPG (**R**eport **P**rogram **G**enerator) is a language developed for basic business applications. Its main function is the efficient preparation of business reports.

MUMPS (**M**assachusetts General Hospital **U**tility **M**ulti**P**rogramming **S**ystem) was one of the first programming languages developed for health care applications. MUMPS allows for the processing of large volumes of data.

C, produced by Bell Laboratories, was used to develop the UNIX operating system. It is a very popular program for system programmers and software designers.

There are three programming languages, LISP, PROLOG, and LOGO, that have been utilized in the development of artifical intelligence and expert systems.

LISP is a programming language developed in 1958 at Massachusetts Institute of Technology by John McCarty. It is designed to process nonnumeric data and is an interactive program.

PROLOG (PROgramming in LOGic) was developed by Allan Colmerauer at the University of Marseilles. The Japanese are using PROLOG as the language of choice for their work in artificial intelligence. Currently this language is beginning to receive more attention in the United States.

LOGO was developed by Seymour Papert and colleagues at the MIT Artificial Intelligence Laboratory. In addition to its applications in artifical intelligence it is now being used in educational programs to teach programming principles to children. LOGO is capable of producing graphics through the use of an interactive input device called a turtle.

ABCs of Choosing a Programming Language

Many considerations go into a decision about which language to use for a particular data processing task. However the answers to the following questions concerning accessibility, background, and compatibility aid in choosing a programming language.

Accessibility. What programming languages are available to you or your organization?

Background. What programming languages are you or your organization's programmer most skilled in working with?

Compatibility. What are any hardware restrictions on the type of languages adaptable to the available computer systems? What type of language is most ideally suited to the particular data processing application?

Answers to these questions will give fundamental guidelines from which to choose the most appropriate language to meet your needs.

Index